ADVANCES IN

Cardiac Surgery®

VOLUME 11

ADVANCES IN

Cardiac Surgery®

VOLUMES 1 THROUGH 8 (OUT OF PRINT)

ADVANCES IN

Cardiac Surgery®

VOLUME 11

Editor-in-Chief
Robert B. Karp, M.D.
Professor of Surgery, Chief of Cardiac Surgery, University of Chicago,
Pritzker School of Medicine, Chicago, Illinois

Editorial Board
Hillel Laks, M.D.
Professor and Chief, Division of Cardiothoracic Surgery; Director, Heart
and Heart–Lung Transplant Program, UCLA Medical Center, Los
Angeles, California

Andrew S. Wechsler, M.D.
Professor and Chairman, Department of Cardiothoracic Surgery,
Allegheny University of the Health Sciences, MCP Hahnemann School
of Medicine, Philadelphia, Pennsylvania

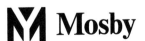 Mosby

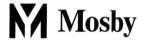

Publisher: Theresa Van Schaik
Associate Publisher: Cynthia Baudendistel
Developmental Editor: Sarah A. Zagarri
Manager, Periodical Editing: Kirk Swearingen
Production Editor: Stephanie M. Geels
Project Supervisor, Production: Joy Moore
Production Assistant: Laura Bayless

Printed in the United States of America
Printing/binding the by Maple-Vail Book Manufacturing Group

Editorial Office:
Mosby, Inc.
11830 Westline Industrial Drive
St. Louis, MO 63146

International Standard Serial Number: 0889-5074
International Standard Book Number: 0-8151-2728-6

Contributors

Ravi Agarwal, M.S., M.Ch.
Staff Surgeon, Institute of Cardiovascular Diseases, Madras, India

Nancy Bridges, M.D.
Associate Professor of Pediatrics, University of Pennsylvania School of Medicine; Medical Director, Thoracic Organ Transplant and Pulmonary Hypertension Programs, Children's Hospital of Philadelphia, Philadelphia, Pennsylvania

Brian F. Buxton, M.B.M.S., F.R.A.C.S., F.R.C.S.
Professor of Cardiac Surgery, University of Melbourne; Director of Cardiac Surgery, Austin and Repatriation Medical Centre, Melbourne, Victoria, Australia

K.M. Cherian, M.S., F.R.A.C.S.
Professor Emeritus, M.G.R. Medical University; Director and Chief of Cardiac Surgery, Institute of Cardiovascular Diseases, Madras, India

Ray Chu-Jeng Chiu, M.D., Ph.D.
Professor and Chairman, Division of Cardiothoracic Surgery, McGill University; Director, Division of Cardiothoracic Surgery, McGill University Health Centre, Montreal, Quebec, Canada

Tirone E. David, M.D.
Professor of Surgery, University of Toronto; Head, Division of Cardiovascular Surgery, The Toronto Hospital, Toronto, Ontario, Canada

John A. Fuller, M.B.B.S., F.R.A.C.P., F.R.C.P.(Edin)
Chief of Perfusion, Epworth Hospital, Melbourne, Victoria, Australia

Charles B. Huddleston, M.D.
Associate Professor of Surgery, Division of Cardiothoracic Surgery, Department of Surgery, Washington University School of Medicine; Chief, Pediatric Cardiothoracic Surgery, St. Louis Children's Hospital, St. Louis, Missouri

Hillel Laks, M.D.
Professor and Chief, Division of Cardiothoracic Surgery; Director, Heart and Heart–Lung Transplant Program, UCLA Medical Center, Los Angeles, California

Daniel Marelli, M.D.
Assistant Clinical Professor, Division of Cardiothoracic Surgery, UCLA School of Medicine, Los Angeles, California

Eric N. Mendeloff, M.D.
Assistant Professor of Surgery, Division of Cardiothoracic Surgery, Department of Surgery, Washington University School of Medicine; Attending Pediatric Cardiothoracic Surgeon, St. Louis Children's Hospital, St. Louis, Missouri

Jonah Odim, M.D., Ph.D., F.R.C.S.(C.)
Division of Cardiothoracic Surgery, UCLA School of Medicine, UCLA Medical Center, Los Angeles, California

Albert J. Pfister, M.D.
Assistant Clinical Professor in Surgery, The George Washington University School of Medicine; Senior Attending Surgeon, Washington Hospital Center, Washington, D.C.

Alistair G. Royse, M.B.B.S., F.R.A.C.S.
Surgical Associate and Examiner, University of Melbourne; Cardiothoracic Surgeon, Royal Melbourne Hospital, Melbourne, Victoria, Australia

N. Madhu Sankar, M.S., Ph.D., D.N.B.
Consultant Cardiac Surgeon, Institute of Cardiovascular Diseases, Madras, India

Richard J. Shemin, M.D.
Professor of Surgery, Boston University School of Medicine; Chairman, Department of Cardiovascular Surgery, Vice Chairman, Division of Surgery, Boston Medical Center, Boston, Massachusetts

James Tatoulis, M.B.B.S., F.R.A.C.S.
Senior Academic Associate, University of Melbourne; Director of Cardiac Surgery, Royal Melbourne Hospital, Melbourne, Victoria, Australia

Christo I. Tchervenkov, M.D., F.R.C.S.C.
Associate Professor of Surgery, McGill University; Director of Cardiovascular Surgery, Montreal Children's Hospital of the McGill University Health Centre, Montreal, Quebec, Canada

John C. Tsang, M.D.
Chief Cardiothoracic Surgery Resident, Montreal Children's Hospital of the McGill University Health Centre, Montreal, Quebec, Canada

Contents

4. Cardiac Cell Transplantation: The Autologous Skeletal Myoblast Implantation for Myocardial Regeneration

C HAPTER 1

Randomized Studies of Coronary Artery Bypass Grafting vs. Medical or Percutaneous Catheter-based Revascularization: A Review

Richard J. Shemin, M.D.
Professor of Surgery, Boston University School of Medicine; Chairman, Department of Cardiovascular Surgery, Vice Chairman, Division of Surgery, Boston Medical Center, Boston, Massachusetts

The treatment of coronary artery disease (CAD) has evolved as our understanding of the pathology and mechanisms of disease have improved. However, the development and implementation of the coronary artery bypass (CABG) operation and later direct catheter-based interventions (percutaneous transluminal coronary angioplasty [PTCA], atherectomy, and stents) have been revolutionary.[1,2] These are among the most commonly performed medical procedures, at considerable expense, aimed at relieving the symptoms and improving survival for the disease that remains the most common cause of death in adults in most of the developed Western World, especially the United States. During 1994 in the United States, more than 480,000 PTCA and 501,000 CABG procedures were performed.[3]

As we enter the next millenium with a growing population and an explosion of the "baby boomer" population into the elderly segment of the population, the impact of CAD is projected to be ever greater. The economic pressures on our health care expenditures, especially the Medicare program, demand that we understand through evidence-based research the appropriate role of these procedures to prevent their costly and indiscriminately wasteful application.

This chapter is intended to present the published data comparing CABG, PTCA, and medical therapy. Clinical trials are the gold standard but have their limitations. They have been performed on specific patient subgroups during the past 20 years, making their data's applicability to current medical and surgical practice often challenging. However, a thorough understanding of the data is mandatory for the modern physician or surgeon to base decisions for patients on information derived from evidence-based studies.

Medical therapy has made significant advances since the early trials comparing medical and surgical therapy performed in the 1970s. Routine treatment with aspirin, β-blockers for secondary prophylaxis after a myocardial infarction (MI), use of angiotensin-converting enzyme inhibitors for heart failure or left ventricular (LV) dysfunction, and addition of calcium channel blockers to nitrates and β-blockers for angina relief have been among the many advances in medical therapy that reduce symptoms and often improve mortality. The control of risk factors such as blood pressure, smoking, body weight, exercise, lipid profile, and diabetes is fundamental to all patients with established CAD or with risk factors, especially a family history of CAD. When myocardial revascularization is considered, the goals are to (1) alleviate symptoms, (2) improve survival, or (3) prevent nonfatal cardiovascular events, such as congestive heart failure and MI.

Within the first decade of the development and perfection of the technique of CABG surgery, three major randomized trials were launched to compare CABG with medical therapy. Myocardial preservation during CABG surgery was under active investigation. Therefore, the operative mortality rates were much greater, especially in higher risk groups (e.g., LV dysfunction), than are currently expected with CABG surgery. In addition, all of these studies were in a surgical era before the routine use of the internal thoracic artery, standardization of techniques for myocardial protection, or the routine use of aspirin to improve vein graft patency. The Veterans Administration (VA) Coronary Artery Bypass Surgery Cooperative Study, the European Coronary Surgery Study (ECSS), the Coronary Artery Surgery Study (CASS), and the associated trial registries have shaped current therapy by clearly showing that the absolute mortality benefit of CABG is proportional to the long-term risk of medical therapy (Table 1).[4-17]

From 1972 to 1974, the VA trial randomized 686 men with stable angina and more than 50% stenosis in at least one major coronary artery. Two high-risk subgroups were identified: high-risk

TABLE 1.

Patient Characteristics and Results From Three Randomized Trials of CABG vs. Medical Therapy

Characteristic	VA	CASS	ECSS
n	686	780	768
Date	1972-1974	1974-1979	1973-1976
Age (yr)	No limit	≤65	<65
% Male	100	90	100
Diseased vessels	≥1	≥1	≥2
Angina class			
Asymptomatic	0	26	0
Class III-IV	58	0	42
Lesion requirement	≥50%	≥70%	≥50%
Ejection fraction	≥25%	≥35%	≥50%
Operative mortality	5.8%	1.4%	3.3%
Improved CABG survival	1. Left main up to 11 years 2. High angiographic risk group up to 11 years 3. High clinical risk group up to 11 years	1. LVEF ≤ 50% especially with 3VD at 10 years	1. Significant 3VD at 12 years 2. 2VD with proximal > 50% LAD stenosis at 12 years

Abbreviations: CABG, coronary artery bypass graft; *VA,* Veterans Administration; *CASS,* Coronary Artery Surgery Study; *ECSS,* European Coronary Surgery Study; *LVEF,* left ventricular ejection fraction; *VD,* vessel disease; *LAD,* left anterior descending artery.

angiographic (3-vessel disease and LV dysfunction, with an ejection fraction [EF] of less than 50%) and high-risk clinical (two or more of the following: resting ECG ST depression, history of MI, history of hypertension). The entire study population has been followed up with published results at 18 years.[5] Survival benefit for surgery was demonstrated at year 7 but not at years 5, 11, 15, or 18 for the entire study population. The subgroup with left main disease had significantly improved survival up to 7 years. Excluding patients with left main disease, survival did not differ with medical therapy up to 11 years' follow-up. Subgroups, excluding those with left main disease, with high clinical or angiographic risk had a significant survival advantage with CABG for 11 years; thereafter survival was the same. Regarding relief of angina, surgical treatment was significantly better among all patients at 5 years. Graft clo-

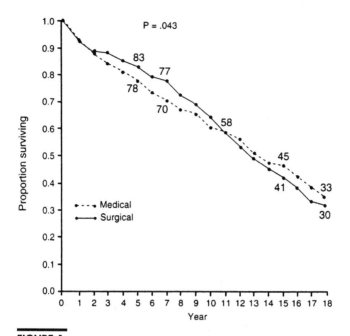

FIGURE 1.
Veterans Administration Coronary Artery Bypass Surgery Cooperative
Study survival rates for all patients. (Courtesy of the VA Coronary Artery
Bypass Surgery Cooperative Study Group: Eighteen-year follow-up in the
Veterans Affairs Cooperative Study of Coronary Artery Bypass Surgery for
stable angina. *Circulation* 86[1]:123-125, 1992.)

sure rates were 29%, 36%, and 50%, respectively, at 1, 5, and 10
years postoperatively. Therefore, the VA trial has shaped current
decision making by identifying patients with left main disease, 3-
vessel disease with LV dysfunction (EF < 50%), and those at clinically high risk as having a survival advantage with surgical therapy
up to 11 years; thereafter progression of disease and vein graft disease neutralized the surgical advantage (Figs 1, 2, and 3).

From 1974 to 1979, the CASS trial randomized 780 patients with
mild, stable angina pectoris to medical therapy or CABG.[8] Patients
with left main disease and those with an EF of less than 35% were
excluded from randomization. At the 5- and 10-year follow-up, no
significant survival advantage was found. However, the surgical
and medical mortalities were very low. Subgroup studies clearly
identified a CABG survival advantage for patients with 3-vessel disease and an LV EF of less than 50% at 10 years (Figs 4 and 5).

From 1973 to 1976, the ECSS randomized 768 men with 2- and 3-
vessel disease (with significant angina pectoris) and preserved LV
function (LV EF > 50%) to medical therapy or CABG. Trial results at
5, 10, and 12 years of follow-up demonstrated a survival advantage

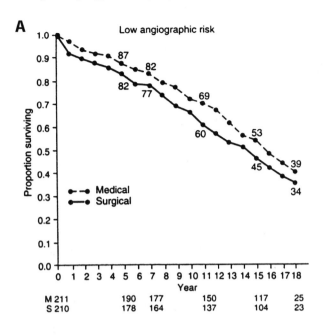

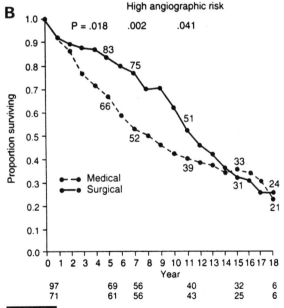

FIGURE 2.
Veterans Administration Coronary Artery Bypass Surgery Cooperative
Study. Cumulative survival rates for patients with low **(A)** and high **(B)**
angiographic risk. (Courtesy of the VA Coronary Artery Bypass Surgery
Cooperative Study Group: Eighteen-year follow-up in the Veterans Affairs
Cooperative Study of Coronary Artery Bypass Surgery for stable angina.
Circulation 86[1]:123-125, 1992.)

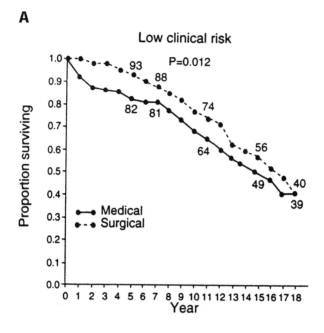

A

Low clinical risk

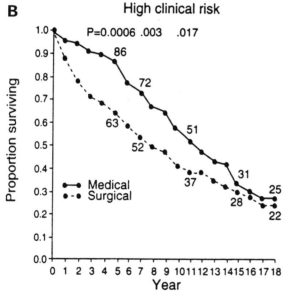

B

High clinical risk

FIGURE 3.
Veterans Administration Coronary Artery Bypass Surgery Cooperative Study. Cumulative survival for patients with low **(A)** and high **(B)** clinical risk. (Courtesy of the VA Coronary Artery Bypass Surgery Cooperative Study Group: Eighteen-year follow-up in the Veterans Affairs Cooperative Study of Coronary Artery Bypass Surgery for stable angina. *Circulation* 86[1]:123-125, 1992.)

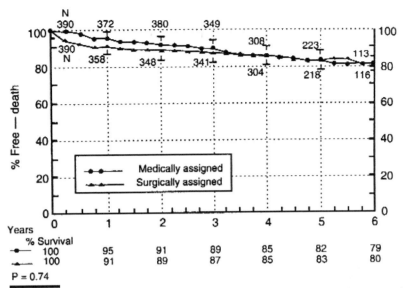

FIGURE 4.
Coronary Artery Surgery Study (CASS). Freedom from death and myocardial infarction for medical and surgical groups. (Reprinted by permission of *The New England Journal of Medicine,* from Myocardial infarction and mortality in the coronary artery surgery study [CASS] randomized trial. *N Engl J Med* 310:750-758. Copyright 1984, Massachusetts Medical Society. All rights reserved.)

for the patients who had CABG performed. Subgroup analysis of patients with 2-vessel disease showed no survival advantage between medical or surgical therapy. However, patients with 2-vessel disease in which one of the lesions involved a 50% proximal stenosis of the left anterior descending (LAD) coronary artery had a survival advantage with CABG. The subgroup of patients with 3-vessel disease also had a significant survival advantage (Figs 6, 7, and 8).[4]

These three major trials consistently documented the superb relief of anginal symptoms, improved activity levels, and reduction in medications afforded the CABG patients. The CABG procedure and its palliation was time limited because of progression of disease involving native coronary arteries and vein graft disease.

The limitations of these trials' results to current practice should be understood. The trials were confined mainly to patients younger than 65 years. Presently, more than half of most current series are inpatients older than 65 years. Only CASS included women and had patients in whom the internal thoracic artery was used (14% of patients) as a conduit. There was no concerted attempt to control lipid levels after randomization, and aspirin was not used in either medical or surgical patients. High-risk patients were in the minority in these trials. In spite of these limitations, certain baseline

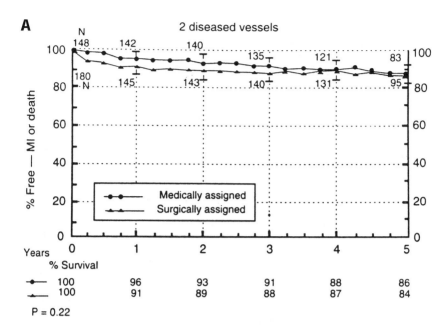

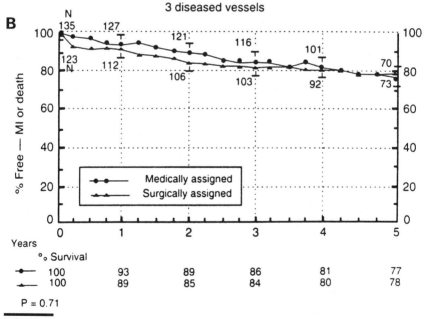

FIGURE 5.
Coronary Artery Surgery Study (CASS). Survival and absence of myocardial infarction *(MI)* with 2-vessel **(A)** and 3-vessel **(B)** disease. (Reprinted by permission of *The New England Journal of Medicine,* from Myocardial infarction and mortality in the coronary artery surgery study [CASS] randomized trial. *N Engl J Med* 310:750-758. Copyright 1984, Massachusetts Medical Society. All rights reserved.)

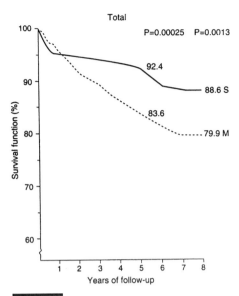

FIGURE 6.
European Coronary Surgery Study (ECSS) survival in the total population. *Abbreviations: M,* medical group; *S,* surgical group. (Courtesy of European Coronary Surgery Study Group: Long-term results of prospective randomized study of coronary artery bypass surgery in stable angina pectoris. *Lancet* 2[8309]:1173-1180. Copyright 1982, The Lancet Ltd.)

anatomical and physiologic risk factors for survival (e.g., left main disease, number of diseased vessels, involvement of the proximal LAD, global LV dysfunction, and degree of ischemia) were identified. Furthermore, the greater the baseline risk for medical mortality, the greater the surgical benefit over medical therapy.

Attempts to overcome the inherent limitation of small numbers of patients who underwent randomization in each trial have led to a meta-analysis of the three major trials plus four minor trials, resulting in a total of 2,649 patients randomly assigned to either CABG or medical therapy during the 1970s and early 1980s. These patients primarily had chronic stable angina and mostly were men between 40 and 60 years of age.[7] The surgical mortality rate was less than the medical mortality rate at 5 years (10.23% vs. 15.8%, relative risk [RR] 0.61), 7 years (10.2% vs. 21.7%, RR 0.68), and 10 years (26.4% vs. 30.5%, RR 0.83). At 10 years, 40% of the patients who had been randomly assigned to medical therapy had crossed over to CABG. Such crossovers always tend to underestimate the real CABG benefits, especially in high-risk groups. Over time, the CABG net benefit was not seen for 2 to 3 years because in a prophylactic surgical treatment trial, the impact of perioperative mortality requires the involved patients to survive long enough to

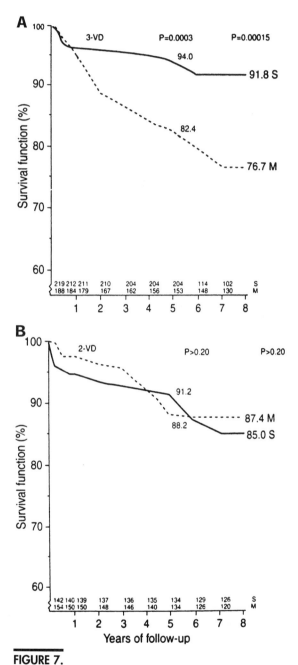

FIGURE 7.
European Coronary Surgery Study (ECSS) survival curves. Medical *(M)* vs. surgical *(S)* groups with 3-vessel disease *(3-VD)* **(A)** and with 2-VD **(B)**. (Courtesy of European Coronary Surgery Study Group: Long-term results of prospective randomized study of coronary artery bypass surgery in stable angina pectoris. *Lancet* 2[8309]:1173-1180. Copyright 1982, The Lancet Ltd.)

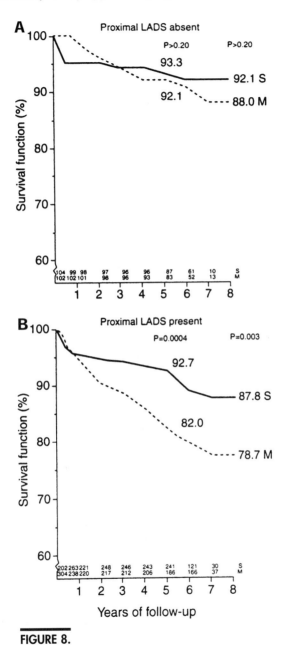

FIGURE 8.
European Coronary Surgery Study (ECSS) survival curves in patients with 2-vessel disease without **(A)** and with **(B)** proximal left anterior descending *(LAD)* coronary artery involvement. *Abbreviations: M,* medical group; *S,* surgical group. (Courtesy of European Coronary Surgery Study Group: Long-term results of prospective randomized study of coronary artery bypass surgery in stable angina pectoris. *Lancet* 2[8309]:1173-1180. Copyright 1982, The Lancet Ltd.)

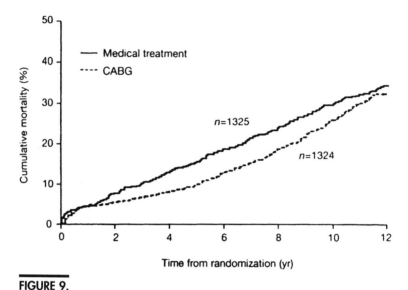

FIGURE 9.
Meta-analysis results of overall survival of the medical and surgically randomized patients. *Abbreviation: CABG,* coronary artery bypass graft. (Courtesy of Yusuf S, Zucker D, Peduzzi P, et al: Effect of coronary artery bypass graft surgery on survival: Overview of 10-year results from randomised trials by the Coronary Artery Bypass Graft Surgery Trialists Collaboration. *Lancet* 344[8922]:563-570. Copyright 1994, The Lancet Ltd.)

accrue a net benefit from treatment (Fig 9). The CABG group advantage improved up to 5 to 7 years postoperatively and then narrowed, so that by year 12 the advantage was gone. The loss of surgical benefit clearly is caused by progression of disease and vein graft disease in the surgical patients, but the impact of crossover in the medical group results in an enhanced narrowing of the real-time risk survival curve because crossover medical patients have their late survival enhanced by CABG.[18]

The meta-analysis confirmed the survival advantage of CABG over medical therapy for 3-vessel disease (RR 0.58, $P < 0.001$), left main disease (RR 0.32, $P = 0.004$), and LAD involvement (RR 0.58, $P = 0.001$) even in 1- or 2-vessel disease and regardless of LV function. However, in patients with LV dysfunction vs. those without, the absolute benefit was twice as great. The absolute vs. real-time benefits of CABG are illustrated when medical subgroups with risk scores stratified by clinical and angiographic factors were compared, demonstrating the CABG advantage for high- and moderate-risk medical groups (5-year medical mortality of 23% and 11.5%, respectively). The low-risk medical groups (5-year medical mortality of 5.5%) will not be expected to have the survival benefit but may benefit from surgical relief and reduction in cardiac events (Table 2).

TABLE 2.

Outcomes of Various Subgroups in Medical Therapy *(MT)* vs. CABG Trials at 5 Years

Subgroup	Overall Numbers Deaths	Overall Numbers Patients	MT Mortality Rate (%)	Odds Ratio (95% CI)	P for CABG vs. MT	P for Interaction
Vessel disease	21	271	9.9	0.54 (0.22-1.33)	0.18	0.19
One vessel						
Two vessels	92	859	11.7	0.84 (0.54-1.32)	0.45	
Three vessels	189	1341	17.6	0.58 (0.42-0.80)	<0.001	
Left main artery	39	150	36.5	0.32 (0.15-0.70)	0.004	
No LAD disease	50	606	8.3	1.05 (0.58-1.90)	0.88	0.06
One or two vessels						
Three vessels	46	410	14.5	0.47 (0.25-0.89)	0.02	
Left main artery	16	51	45.8	0.27 (0.08-0.90)	0.03	
Overall	112	1067	12.3	0.66 (0.44-1.00)	0.05	
LAD disease present	63	524	14.6	0.58 (0.34-1.01)	0.05	0.44
One or two vessels						
Three vessels	143	929	19.1	0.61 (0.42-0.88)	0.009	
Left main artery	22	96	32.7	0.30 (0.11-0.84)	0.02	
Overall	228	1549	18.3	0.58 (0.43-0.77)	0.001	
LV function	228	2095	]3.3	0.61 (0.46-0.81)	<0.001	0.90
Normal						
Abnormal	115	549	25.2	0.59 (0.39-0.91)	0.02	

(continued)

TABLE 2. (continued)

Subgroup	Overall Numbers Deaths	Patients	MT Mortality Rate (%)	Odds Ratio (95% CI)	P for CABG vs. MT	P for Interaction
Exercise test status	102	664	17.4	0.69 (0.45-1.07)	0.10	0.37
Missing						
Normal	60	585	11.6	0.78 (0.45-1.35)	0.38	
Abnormal	183	1400	16.8	0.52 (0.37-0.72)	<0.001	
Severity of angina (CCS)						
Class O, I, II	178	1716	12.5	0.63 (0.46-0.87)	0.005	0.69
Class III, IV	167	924	22.4	0.57 (0.40-0.81)	0.001	

Abbreviations: CI, confidence interval; *CABG,* coronary artery bypass graft; *LAD,* left anterior descending artery; *LV,* left ventricular; *CCS,* Canadian Coronary Severity class.

(Courtesy of Yusuf S, Zucker D, Peduzzi P, et al: Effect of coronary artery bypass graft surgery on survival: Overview of 10-year results from randomised trials by the Coronary Artery Bypass Graft Surgery Trialists Collaboration. *Lancet* 344[8922]:563-570. Copyright 1994, The Lancet Ltd.)

Registry studies have shown a favorable impact on subsequent MI in the high-risk group of 3-vessel disease and severe angina.[12] The meta-analysis did not show an overall impact of CABG on subsequent MI partly because of the 10.3% incidence of death or MI in the 30-day perioperative period in the CABG group, even though the 5-year death or MI incidence was 24.4% in the CABG patients and 30% in the medical patients.[7] Unfortunately, the trials did not study rehospitalization, quality of life, or cost. It is reasonable to expect that in the modern CABG era, the positive effect of CABG or even catheter-based interventions may be superior to the data presented. This is suggested by the Asymptomatic Cardiac Ischemia Pilot study, a medical vs. revascularization trial in the current era, in which the revascularization group had significant reductions at 2 years in mortality, late death or MI, recurrence of angina, and need for rehospitalization.[19-21]

Approximately a decade after CABG became the accepted surgical alternative to treat CAD, PTCA emerged. Originally conceived to be an alternative to CABG, in reality the rate of utilization of both procedures has grown. PTCA as an alternative to medical therapy primarily is used to treat single-vessel disease and, more recently, the "culprit lesion" in multivessel disease, the occluded vessel in acute MI, and multiple vessels in multivessel disease.

Because of the high rates of procedural success of both CABG and PTCA in single-vessel disease, it is unclear which procedure is the optimal mode of therapy. Three randomized trials have provided comparative data. A single-center Swiss trial published in 1994 randomly assigned 134 patients with LAD disease to PTCA or CABG with a left internal mammary artery (IMA).[22] During 2.5 years of follow-up, one death occurred in the CABG group and none in the PTCA group. Both groups had equivalent relief of angina (> 95% Canadian Coronary Severity class I at 1 year) and equivalent results on exercise testing. The only difference was a 34% rate of repeat revascularization in the PTCA group because of restenosis. Similar results were found in the British RITA[23] and Brazilian MASS studies.[24] Pocock et al.[25] performed a meta-analysis with similar conclusions. Therefore, both PTCA and CABG are highly effective for single-vessel LAD disease in relieving symptoms. Neither procedure unequivocally reduces mortality rate or occurrence of MI. The perception that PTCA is simple to perform, reduces invasiveness, and is less costly than CABG is tarnished by the need to perform repeat PTCA procedures. In addition, the advent of MID CAB (minimally invasive directed coronary artery bypass) further reduces the invasive nature of CABG for single-vessel disease, preserves the ability to use the internal thoracic artery, and reduces hospital cost, recovery time, and time away from work. These facts, coupled with the results from a meta-analysis of CABG vs. medical therapy for 1- to 2-vessel disease with proximal LAD lesions, which showed a surgical survival advantage, should be considered when choosing a procedure for a patient. Even though in current practice usually the PTCA or stent is chosen as the therapy of choice, a randomized trial vs. MID CAB with composite end points (because death rates are so low in this group, to adequately power the study the sample size would need to include thousands of patients) should be undertaken.

For multivessel disease, CABG was the standard for moderate- and high-risk subgroups, severe 2- and 3-vessel disease, and patients with LV dysfunction. There have been nine published clinical trials comparing PTCA with CABG that are broadly comparable but heterogeneous in design, methods, and follow-up. Five trials were single center and four were multicenter. The main characteristics of these trials are summarized in Table 3. The results and conclusions of these trials are similar with a few specific caveats. In addition, the meta-analysis of all the trials combined (except the Bypass Angioplasty Revascularization Investigation [BARI], which had not yet published its 5-year data when the meta-analysis by Pocock et al.[25] was published) helps in comparing the trials. The major trials were BARI,[26] Coronary Angioplasty vs. Bypass Revascularization Investigation (CABRI),[27] Emory Angioplasty vs. Surgery Trial (EAST),[28] Argentine Randomized Trial of PTCA vs. CABG in Multivessel Disease (ERACI), German Angioplasty Bypass Surgery Investigation (GABI),[29] Randomized Intervention Treatment of Angina (RITA),[23] Swiss, and Toulouse trials.[7]

In the CABRI trial, 1,054 patients who had symptomatic 2-vessel (57%) or 3-vessel (42%) disease and were aged 75 years or younger underwent randomization. Most patients had a normal EF (65%). Some had impaired (25%) LV function. The total mortality rate was 3.9% for PTCA and 2.7% for CABG at 1 year ($P = 0.30$) and was still not significantly different at 65 months ($P = 0.068$). The risk of nonfatal MI after PTCA and CABG was similar ($P = 0.23$). In the PTCA group during the first year of follow-up, 33.6% of patients required repeat revascularization ($P < 0.001$), and use of antianginal medication was increased($P < 0.001$) (Fig 10).[27]

In the EAST trial, 392 patients with 2- or 3-vessel disease (only 7.7% of those screened) underwent randomization. The IMA was used in 90% of CABG patients. The 3-year overall mortality was 6.2% for CABG and 7.1% for PTCA ($P = 0.73$). Q-wave MI was 19.6% for CABG vs. 14.6% for PTCA (P = 0.21). Large residual thallium deficits were detected in 5.7% of patients who had CABG vs. 9.6% of patients who had PTCA ($P = 0.17$). The repeat revascularization rate was 13% in the CABG group vs. 54% in the PTCA group ($P < 0.001$) (Figs 11 and 12).[28]

TABLE 3.
Main Characteristics of 9 Prospective, Randomized Trials of PTCA vs. CABG[40]

	BARI	CABRI	EAST	ERACI	GABI	MASS	RITA	Swiss	Toulouse
Location	North America, multicenter	Europe, multicenter	Emory University (Atlanta, GA), single-center	Argentina, single-center	Germany, multicenter	Brazil, single-center	Britain, multicenter	Switzerland, single-center	France, single-center
Patients screened (n)	25 200	?	5118	1409	8981	?	17 237	?	?
Random-ized (%)	1829 (7.3)	1054	392 (7.7)	127 (9.0)	359 (4.0)	214	1011 (4.8)	142	152
Equivalent revascu-larization required	No	No	No	No	Yes	Yes	Yes	Yes	Yes
Follow-up Planned duration (yr)	10	5-10	3	3	1	3.5	5	2.5	3
Completed	No	No	Yes	Yes	Yes	Yes	No	Yes	Yes

(continued)

TABLE 3. (continued)

	BARI	CABRI	EAST	ERACI	GABI	MASS	RITA	Swiss	Toulouse
Primary endpoint	Mortality, MI	Mortality, nonfatal MI, angina, functional capacity	Combined death, MI, and large thallium defect	Combined death, MI, and angina	Freedom from angina at 1 year (> CCS 2)	Combined cardiac death, MI, refractory angina	Combined death and MI	Death, MI, repeat revascularization	?
No. of stenotic vessels (%)									
One	0	0	0	0	0	100	45	100	—
Two	56	58	60	55	81	—	43	—	49
Three	43	40	40	45	19	—	12	—	14
Mean ejection fraction (%)	58	63	61	61	?	75	?	?	?
Average age (yr)	61	61	62	57	59	56	57	56	?

CCS class 3 or 4 angina (%)	?	65	80	?	65	?	60	89	?
Mammary artery used [% of CABG procedures]	82	?	90	77	37	100	74	100	?
Male/female	74:26	63:37	74:26	54:46	80:20	58:42	81:19	80:20	?
Previous MI (%)	?	41	41	32	47	?	43	0	?

Abbreviations: PTCA, percutaneous transluminal coronary angioplasty; CABG, coronary artery bypass graft; BARI, Bypass Angioplasty Revascularization Investigation; CABRI, Coronary Angioplasty vs. Bypass Revascularization Investigation; EAST, Emory Angioplasty vs. Surgery Trial; ERACI, Argentine Randomized Trial of PTCA vs. CABG in Multivessel Disease; GABI, German Angioplasty Bypass Surgery Investigation; MASS, Medicine, Angioplasty or Surgery Study; RITA, Randomized Intervention Treatment of Angina; MI, myocardial infarction; CCS, Canadian Coronary Severity.

(Courtesy of Raco D, Rihal CS, Yusuf S: Randomized trials of percutaneous transluminal coronary angioplasty: Comparison of medical and surgical therapy, in Grech ED, Ramsdale DR [eds]: *Practical Interventional Cardiology.* St Louis, Mosby, 1977, p 323.

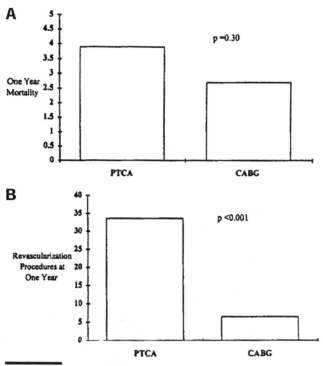

FIGURE 10.
Coronary Angioplasty vs. Bypass Revascularization Investigation (CABRI). **A,** 1-year percutaneous transluminal coronary angioplasty *(PTCA)* vs. coronary artery bypass graft *(CABG)* mortality. **B,** 1-year PTCA vs. CABG repeat revascularization rates.

In the ERACI trial, 127 patients underwent randomization (only 9% of those screened). The IMA was used in 77% of CABG patients. The in-hospital complication rates and 1-year death and MI rates were not statistically different. The PTCA group had a marked increased incidence of angina and need for repeat procedures (32.2% PTCA vs. 3.3% CABG [P < 0.001]) (Fig 13).[30]

In the GABI trial, 359 patients underwent randomization (only 4% of those screened). Only 37% of patients in the surgical group received an IMA graft. Periprocedural Q-wave MI was 8.1% for CABG vs. 2.3% for PTCA *(P* = 0.22). At 1 year, freedom from angina was 74% for CABG group vs. 71% for PTCA group. The composite death or MI end point (including periprocedural MI) was 13.6% for CABG vs. 6% for PTCA *(P* = 0.017). Repeat interventions were 23% repeat PTCA and 18% CABG in the patients initially randomly assigned to PTCA. In the initial CABG group, only 1% underwent repeat CABG and 5% a subsequent PTCA. Patients who underwent CABG had a reduced medication (antianginal) require-

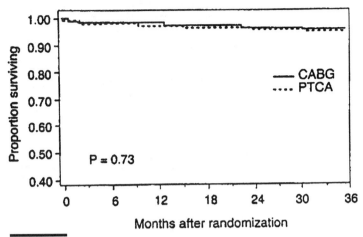

FIGURE 11.
Emory Angioplasty vs. Surgery Trial (EAST). Coronary artery bypass graft *(CABG)* vs. percutaneous transluminal coronary angioplasty *(PTCA)* 3-year survival curves. (Reprinted by permission of *The New England Journal of Medicine,* from King SB III, Lembo NJ, Weintraub WS, et al: A randomized trial comparing coronary angioplasty with coronary bypass surgery: Emory Angioplasty versus Surgery Trial [EAST]. *N Engl J Med* 331:1044-1050. Copyright 1994, Massachusetts Medical Society. All rights reserved.)

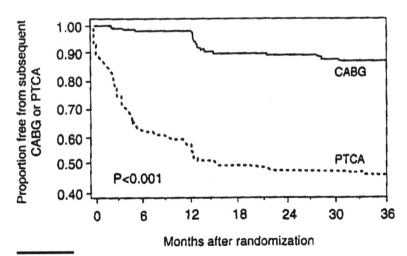

FIGURE 12.
Emory Angioplasty vs. Surgery Trial (EAST). Coronary artery bypass graft *(CABG)* vs. percutaneous transluminal coronary angioplasty *(PTCA)* repeat revascularization curves. (Reprinted by permission of *The New England Journal of Medicine,* from King SB III, Lembo NJ, Weintraub WS, et al: A randomized trial comparing coronary angioplasty with coronary bypass surgery: Emory Angioplasty versus Surgery Trial [EAST]. *N Engl J Med* 331:1044-1050. Copyright 1994, Massachusetts Medical Society. All rights reserved.)

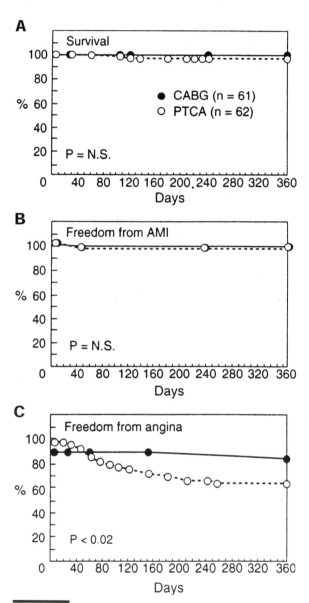

FIGURE 13.
Argentine Randomized Trial of PTCA vs. CABG in Multivessel Disease
(ERACI). **A,** survival. **B,** freedom from acute myocardial infarction *(AMI).* **C,**
freedom from angina. *Abbreviations: CABG,* coronary artery bypass graft;
PTCA, percutaneous transluminal coronary angioplasty; *N.S.,* not significant.
(Reprinted with permission from the American College of Cardiology, from
Rodriguez A, Boullon F, Perez-Balino N, et al: Argentine Randomized Trial of
Percutaneous Transluminal Coronary Angioplasty Versus Coronary Artery
Bypass Surgery in Multivessel Disease [ERACI]: In-hospital results and 1-year
follow-up. ERACI group. *J Am Coll Cardiol* 22:1060-1067, 1993.)

ment. At 6-month angiography, 13% of vein grafts were occluded and 7% of IMA grafts were nonfunctional, whereas 16% of vessels in which angioplasty had been performed were occluded or restenosed (>70% stenosis) (Fig 14).[29]

In the RITA trial, 1,011 patients underwent randomization (4.8% of those screened). The IMA was used in 74% of CABG patients. At 2.5 years, total mortality was 3.1% for the PTCA group vs. 3.6% for the CABG group (*P* = NS). Combined end points were 9.8% for PTCA vs. 8.6% for CABG (*P* = 0.47). Repeat revascularization was 28.2% in the PTCA patients vs. 2.4% in the CABG group. More PTCA patients required antianginal therapy than did CABG patients (61% vs. 34%) (Fig 15).[23]

In the BARI trial, the most patients (1,829 patients) underwent randomization (still only 7.3% of those screened). The IMA was used in 82% of the surgical patients. The BARI trial had the longest designed period of follow-up (5 years). Mortality was 10.7% in patients who had CABG and 13.7% in those who had PTCA (*P* = 0.19). The incidence of death or Q-wave MI by 5 years was 19.4% for the CABG group vs. 21.3% for the PTCA group. Additional revascularization was performed in 54% of the PTCA patients and 8% of the CABG group. A major subgroup, "treated (oral or insulin agents) diabetics," had a highly significant mortality difference favoring CABG (5-year mortality, 19.4% CABG vs. 34.5% PTCA; *P* = 0.003). The 7-year BARI follow-up data for the primary end point of mortality show a clear statistical benefit for the patients randomly assigned to CABG. Further analysis demonstrates that the difference is attributed to the diabetic population in the BARI trial (Fig 16).[26,31]

BARI substudies showed PTCA and CABG to have similar beneficial effects in regards to quality of life and return to employment. The cost analysis shows that at 3 to 5 years the costs are equivalent, because CABG is associated with more complete revascularization and minimal need for repeat procedures over 5 to 7 years of follow-up (Fig 17).[32]

The meta-analysis of these trials (excluding BARI) by Pocock et al.[25,33] included 3,371 patients. At 2.7 years, mortality was 4.4% for the CABG group vs. 4.6% for the PTCA group (RR 1.08; 95% confidence interval [CI], 0.79-1.50); death or MI was 7.6% for CABG vs. 7.9% for PTCA (RR 1.10; 95% CI, 0.89-1.37). Repeat revascularization was 33.7% for PTCA patients (18% of which were CABG) vs. only 3.3% in the randomized CABG group (*P* < 0.0001) (Figs 18 and 19).

In total, the nine trials have randomly assigned 5,200 patients with multivessel disease to either PTCA or CABG.[25,33,34] The randomized patients are only a fraction of the total number of patients

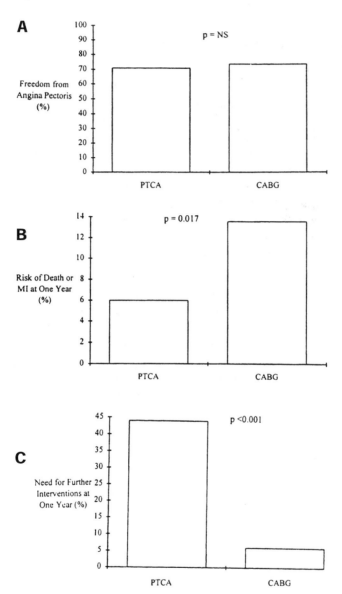

FIGURE 14.

German Angioplasty Bypass Surgery Investigation (GABI): coronary artery
bypass graft *(CABG)* vs. percutaneous transluminal coronary angioplasty
(PTCA). **A,** freedom from angina. **B,** death or myocardial infarction *(MI)* at
1 year. **C,** repeat revascularization. *Abbreviation: NS,* not significant.
(Reprinted by permission of *The New England Journal of Medicine,* from
Hamm C, Reimers J, Ischinger T, et al: A randomized study of coronary
angioplasty compared with bypass surgery in patients with symptomatic
multivessel coronary disease. *N Engl J Med* 331:1037-1043. Copyright
1994, Massachusetts Medical Society. All rights reserved.)

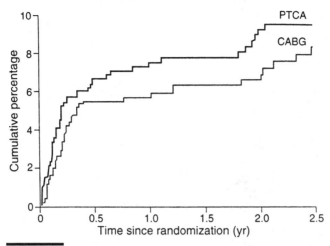

FIGURE 15.
Randomized Intervention Treatment of Angina (RITA). Cumulative risk of death or MI for the CABG and PTCA groups. *Abbreviations: MI,* myocardial infarction; *CABG,* coronary artery bypass graft; *PTCA,* percutaneous transluminal coronary angioplasty. (Courtesy of RITA Trial participants: Coronary angioplasty versus coronary artery bypass surgery: The Randomised Intervention Treatment of Angina [RITA] trial. *Lancet* 341[8845]:573-580. Copyright 1993, The Lancet Ltd.

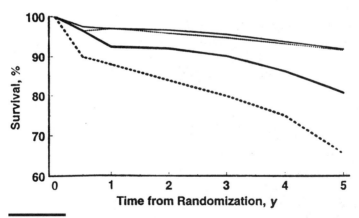

FIGURE 16.
Bypass Angioplasty Revascularization Investigation (BARI). Five-year survival curve for CABG *(solid line)* and PTCA *(dotted line). Upper two curves* represent nondiabetic patients. *Lower two curves* represent treated diabetic patients. (Reprinted by permission of *The New England Journal of Medicine,* from Hamm C, Reimers J, Ischinger T, et al: A randomized study of coronary angioplasty compared with bypass surgery in patients with symptomatic multivessel coronary disease. *N Engl J Med* 331:1037-1043. Copyright 1994, Massachusetts Medical Society. All rights reserved.)

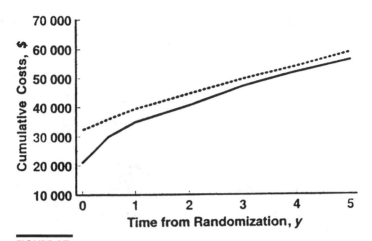

FIGURE 17.
Bypass Angioplasty Revascularization Investigation (BARI). Cumulative costs over time for the CABG *(solid line)* and the PTCA *(dotted line)*. (Reprinted by permission of *The New England Journal of Medicine*, from Hlatky MA, Rogers WJ, Johnstone I, et al: Medical care costs and quality of life after randomization to coronary angioplasty or coronary bypass surgery. *N Engl J Med* 336[2]:92-99. Copyright 1997, Massachusetts Medical Society. All rights reserved.)

screened in the multivessel disease universe. Except for treated diabetics, a superiority of one procedure over the other regarding mortality or MI has not been demonstrated. Clearly, the PTCA groups consistently have more residual angina and require significant numbers of repeat procedures (approximately 40%) mostly within the first 3 years of follow-up (Fig 20).[31] Restenosis is the major limitation of PTCA, and the future or current impact of stents will help improve PTCA results.

In the current trials, the enrolled patients are few in number and have a low risk for medical mortality, suggesting that the studies are inadequately powered to test for treatment differences. Only BARI enrolled moderate-risk CAD patients, but still 60% of patients only had 2-vessel disease. Among the total of 5,200 randomized patients in all the trials, important high-risk subgroups may have a CABG advantage, but the small number of these patients that underwent randomization will prevent small but important mortality differences from being detected statistically. In addition, the very high crossover rate tends to minimize the impact of initial CABG randomization because the intention-to-treat analysis of the PTCA group has up to 20% of PTCA patients crossing over to CABG within the first 3 years of follow-up.

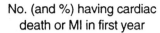

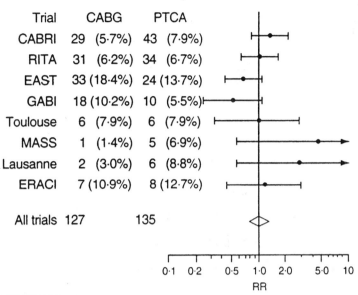

No. (and %) having cardiac
death or MI in first year

Trial	CABG	PTCA
CABRI	29 (5·7%)	43 (7·9%)
RITA	31 (6·2%)	34 (6·7%)
EAST	33 (18·4%)	24 (13·7%)
GABI	18 (10·2%)	10 (5·5%)
Toulouse	6 (7·9%)	6 (7·9%)
MASS	1 (1·4%)	5 (6·9%)
Lausanne	2 (3·0%)	6 (8·8%)
ERACI	7 (10·9%)	8 (12·7%)
All trials	127	135

0·1   0·2   0·5   1·0   2·0   5·0   10
RR

FIGURE 18.
Meta-analysis of coronary artery bypass graft *(CABG)* vs. percutaneous transluminal coronary angioplasty *(PTCA)* trials by Pocock et al. Comparing cardiac death or myocardial infarction *(MI)* at 1 year after procedure. *Abbreviations: CABRI,* Coronary Angioplasty vs. Bypass Revascularization Investigation; *RITA,* Randomized Intervention Treatment of Angina; *EAST,* Emory Angioplasty vs. Surgery Trial; *GABI,* German Angioplasty Bypass Surgery Investigation; *MASS,* Medicine, Angioplasty or Surgery Study; *ERACI,* Argentine Randomized Trial of PTCA vs. CABG in Multivessel Disease; *RR,* relative risk. (Courtesy of Pocock SJ, Henderson RA, Rickards AF, et al: Meta-analysis of randomised trials comparing coronary angioplasty with bypass surgery. *Lancet* 346[8984]:1184-1189. Copyright 1995, The Lancet Ltd.)

Even though randomized clinical trials provide the best data for clinical decisions, it remains useful to supplement this knowledge with information from large observational databases. Duke University Medical Center has long-term survival data for 9,263 patients with angiographically documented disease.[35] These patients were nonrandomly treated, but the prospective follow-up is 97% complete. There are 2,449 medical, 2,924 PTCA, and 3,890 CABG patients. Risk stratification for mortality by angiographic extent of CAD (i.e., number of lesions, proximal LAD location, degree of stenosis [95%, excluding left main less than 75% stenosed]) allowed an organized analysis of CABG, medicine, and PTCA comparisons.

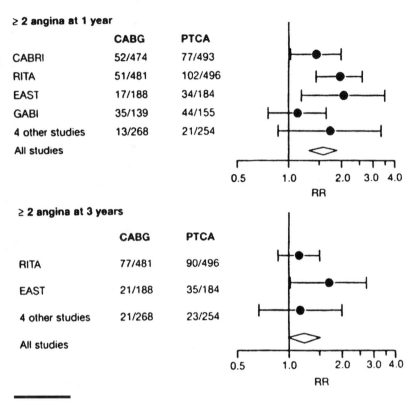

FIGURE 19.
Meta-analysis of coronary artery bypass graft *(CABG)* vs. percutaneous transluminal coronary angioplasty *(PTCA)* trials by Pocock et al. Prevalence of angina at 1 and 3 years after revascularization. *Abbreviations: CABRI,* Coronary Angioplasty vs. Bypass Revascularization Investigation; *RITA,* Randomized Intervention Treatment of Angina; *EAST,* Emory Angioplasty vs. Surgery Trial; *GABI,* German Angioplasty Bypass Surgery Investigation; *RR,* relative risk. (Courtesy of Pocock SJ, Henderson RA, Rickards AF, et al: Meta-analysis of randomised trials comparing coronary angioplasty with bypass surgery. *Lancet* 346[8984]:1184-1189. Copyright 1995, The Lancet Ltd.)

CABG significantly improved long-term patient survival compared with medical therapy for patients with 1- and 2-vessel disease having proximal LAD lesions causing stenosis of greater than 95%, and for all patients with 3-vessel disease (Fig 21). CABG was superior to PTCA in the high-risk strata of 3-vessel disease and 2-vessel disease with proximal LAD lesions causing stenosis of greater than 95%. PTCA was superior to CABG in the low-risk strata (i.e., 1- and 2-vessel disease). The Duke observational data extend the randomized trials and allow further characterization of possible treatment differences. However, the defect of trial design

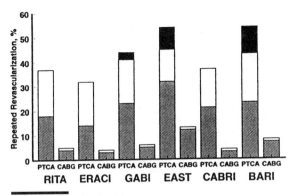

FIGURE 20.
Repeat revascularization risk in 6 randomized PTCA *(white bars)* vs.
CABG *(striped bars)* trials (both = *black bars*). *Abbreviations: PTCA,* per-
cutaneous transluminal coronary angioplasty; *CABG,* coronary artery
bypass graft; *RITA,* Randomized Intervention Treatment of Angina;
ERACI, Argentine Randomized Trial of PTCA vs. CABG in Multivessel
Disease; *GABI,* German Angioplasty Bypass Surgery Investigation; *EAST,*
Emory Angioplasty vs. Surgery Trial; *CABRI,* Coronary Angioplasty vs.
Bypass Revascularization Investigation; *BARI,* Bypass Angioplasty
Revascularization Investigation. (Courtesy of Jones RH, Kesler K, Phillips
HR, et al: Long-term survival benefits of coronary artery bypass grafting
and percutaneous transluminal angioplasty in patients with coronary
artery disease. *J Thorac Cardiovasc Surg* 111:1013-1025, 1996.)

GR	VD	95%	LAD	CABG better Medicine better
1	1	No		
2	1	Yes		
3	2	No		
4	2	Yes		
5	1	Yes	95% Prox	
	2	Yes	95%	
6	2	Yes	95% Prox	
	3	No	Yes	
7	3	Yes	Yes	
8	3	Yes	Prox	
9	3	Yes	95% Prox	

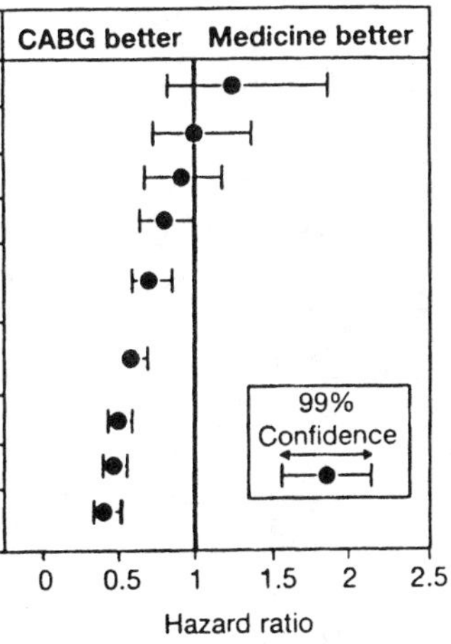

0   0.5   1   1.5   2   2.5
Hazard ratio

FIGURE 21.
Coronary artery bypass graft *(CABG)* vs. medical therapy adjusted hazard
ratios for 9 coronary anatomy groups *(GR)* from the Duke database.
Abbreviations: VD, vessel disease; *LAD,* left anterior descending coronary
artery; *Prox,* proximal; *95%,* degree of coronary stenosis. (Courtesy of Jones
RH, Kesler K, Phillips HR, et al: Long-term survival benefits of coronary artery
bypass grafting and percutaneous transluminal angioplasty in patients with
coronary artery disease. *J Thorac Cardiovasc Surg* 111:1013-1025, 1996.)

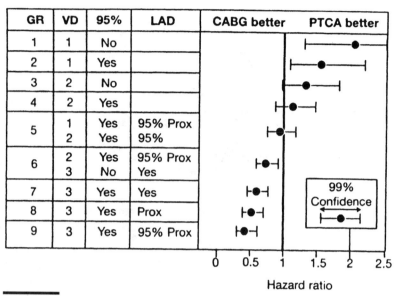

GR	VD	95%	LAD	CABG better	PTCA better
1	1	No			
2	1	Yes			
3	2	No			
4	2	Yes			
5	1	Yes	95% Prox		
	2	Yes	95%		
6	2	Yes	95% Prox		
	3	No	Yes		
7	3	Yes	Yes		
8	3	Yes	Prox		
9	3	Yes	95% Prox		

99% Confidence

Hazard ratio

FIGURE 22.
Coronary artery bypass graft *(CABG)* vs. percutaneous transluminal coronary angioplasty *(PTCA)* for the 9 coronary anatomy groups *(GR)* from the Duke database. *Abbreviations: VD,* vessel disease; *LAD,* left anterior descending coronary artery; *Prox,* proximal; *95%,* degree of coronary stenosis from the Duke database. (Courtesy of Jones RH, Kesler K, Phillips HR, et al: Long-term survival benefits of coronary artery bypass grafting and percutaneous transluminal angioplasty in patients with coronary artery disease. *J Thorac Cardiovasc Surg* 111:1013-1025, 1996.)

and type II errors are best addressed with larger trials that are adequately powered in number of subjects and follow-up times (Fig 22).

The cumulative evidence from trials of myocardial revascularization supports the use of PTCA in low-risk patients and CABG for high-risk patients. Current data cannot determine whether important mortality differences in the order of magnitude of 20% to 30% exist, because the currently completed trials were not powered to deal with this level of difference.[18] CABG clearly provides more complete revascularization, superior angina relief, and superior reduction in mortality in treated diabetics. No differences in MI rates have been seen.

PTCA requires significantly more repeat procedures, and even stents are unlikely to lower this rate to the level of that seen with CABG. Medical cost, patients' quality of life, and the frequency of patients returning to work equalize when both groups are compared within 3 to 5 years of follow-up.[36-39] The advances in CABG surgery and interventional catheter-based procedures will require continued study to ensure that the most appropriate and cost-effective treatment is provided for the patient with CAD. In addition, aggressive institution of medical therapy after myocardial revascularization procedures are performed has great potential to extend life, reduce cardiovascular events, improve quality of life, and control medical costs.

REFERENCES

1. Favaloro RG: Saphenous vein autograft replacement of severe segmental coronary artery occlusion: Operative technique. *Ann Thorac Surg* 5:334-339, 1968.
2. Gruntzig AR, Senning A, Siegenthaler WE: Nonoperative dilatation of coronary artery stenosis: Percutaneous transluminal coronary angioplasty. *N Engl J Med* 301:61-68, 1979.
3. Greaves EJ, Gillum BS: *1994 Summary: National Hospital Discharge Survey. Advance Data From Vital and Health Statistics*, No 278. Hyattsville, Md, National Center for Health Statistics, 1996.
4. European Coronary Surgery Study Group: Long-term results of prospective randomized study of coronary artery bypass surgery in stable angina pectoris. *Lancet* 2:1173-1180, 1982.
5. The VA Coronary Artery Bypass Surgery Cooperative Study Group: Eighteen-year follow-up in the Veterans Affairs Cooperative Study of Coronary Artery Bypass Surgery for stable angina. *Circulation* 86:121-130, 1990.
6. Alderman EL, Bourassa MG, Cohen LS, et al: Ten-year follow-up of survival and myocardial infarction in the randomized Coronary Artery Surgery Study. *Circulation* 82:1629-1646, 1990.
7. Yusuf S, Zucker D, Peduzzi P, et al: Effect of coronary artery bypass graft surgery on survival: Overview of 10-year results from randomised trials by the Coronary Artery Bypass Graft Surgery Trialists Collaboration. *Lancet* 344:563-570, 1994.
8. Coronary Artery Surgery Study (CASS) Principal Investigators and Associates: Myocardial infarction and mortality in the Coronary Artery Surgery Study (CASS) randomized trial. *N Engl J Med* 310:750-758, 1984.
9. Prospective randomised study of coronary artery bypass surgery in stable angina pectoris: Second interim report by the European Coronary Surgery Study Group. *Lancet* 2:491-495, 1980.
10. Caracciolo EA, Davis KB, Sopko G, et al: Comparison of surgical and medical group survival in patients with left main equivalent coronary artery disease: Long-term CASS experience. *Circulation* 91:2335-2344, 1995.
11. Passamani E, Davis KB, Gillespie MJ, et al: A randomized trial of coronary artery bypass surgery: Survival of patients with a low ejection fraction. *N Engl J Med* 312:1665-1671, 1985.
12. Myers WO, Schaff HV, Fisher LD, et al: Time to first new myocardial infarction in patients with severe angina and three-vessel disease comparing medical and early surgical therapy: A CASS registry study of survival. *J Thorac Cardiovasc Surg* 95:382-389, 1988.
13. Eleven-year survival in the Veterans Administration randomized trial

of coronary bypass surgery for stable angina: The Veterans Administration Coronary Artery Bypass Surgery Cooperative Study Group. *N Engl J Med* 311:1333-1339, 1984.

14. Varnauskas E: Twelve-year follow-up of survival in the randomized European Coronary Surgery Study. *N Engl J Med* 319:332-337, 1988.

15. Murphy ML, Hultgren HN, Detre K, et al: Treatment of chronic stable angina: A preliminary report of survival data of the randomized Veterans Administration cooperative study. *N Engl J Med* 297:621-627, 1977.

16. Coronary Artery Surgery Study (CASS): A randomized trial of coronary artery bypass surgery: Survival data. *Circulation* 68:939-950, 1983.

17. Kaiser GC, Davis KB, Fisher LD, et al: Survival following coronary artery bypass grafting in patients with severe angina pectoris (CASS): An observational study. *J Thorac Cardiovasc Surg* 89:513-524, 1985.

18. Solomon AJ, Gersh BJ: Management of chronic stable angina: Medical therapy, percutaneous transluminal coronary angioplasty, and coronary artery bypass graft surgery. Lessons from randomized trials. *Ann Intern Med* 128:216-223, 1998.

19. Chaitman BR, Stone PH, Knatterud GL, et al: Asymptomatic Cardiac Ischemia Pilot (ACIP) study: Impact of anti-ischemia therapy on 12-week rest electrocardiogram and exercise test outcomes. The ACIP Investigators. *J Am Coll Cardiol* 26:585-593, 1995.

20. Rogers WJ, Bourassa MG, Andrews TC, et al: Asymptomatic Cardiac Ischemia Pilot (ACIP) study: Outcome at 1 year for patients with asymptomatic cardiac ischemia randomized to medical therapy or revascularization. The ACIP Investigators. *J Am Coll Cardiol* 26:594-605, 1995.

21. Davies RF, Goldberg AD, Forman S, et al: Asymptomatic Cardiac Ischemia Pilot (ACIP) study two-year follow-up: Outcomes of patients randomized to initial strategies of medical therapy versus revascularization. *Circulation* 95:2037-2043, 1997.

22. Goy JJ, Eeckhout E, Burnand B, et al: Coronary angioplasty versus left internal mammary artery grafting for isolated proximal left anterior descending artery stenosis. *Lancet* 343:1449-1453, 1994.

23. Coronary angioplasty versus coronary artery bypass surgery: The Randomised Intervention Treatment of Angina (RITA) trial. *Lancet* 341:573-580, 1993.

24. Hueb WA, Bellotti G, de Oliveira SA, et al: The Medicine, Angioplasty or Surgery Study (MASS): A prospective, randomized trial of medical therapy, balloon angioplasty or bypass surgery for single proximal left anterior descending artery stenoses. *J Am Coll Cardiol* 26:1600-1605, 1995.

25. Pocock SJ, Henderson RA, Rickards AF, et al: Meta-analysis of randomised trials comparing coronary angioplasty with bypass surgery. *Lancet* 346:1184-1189, 1995.

26. Comparison of coronary bypass surgery with angioplasty in patients with multivessel disease: The Bypass Angioplasty Revascularization Investigation (BARI) Investigators. *N Engl J Med* 335:217-225, 1996.

27. First-year results of CABRI (Coronary Angioplasty Versus Bypass Revascularization Investigation): CABRI Trial Participants. *Lancet* 346:1179-1184, 1995.

28. King SB III, Lembo NJ, Weintraub WS, et al: A randomized trial comparing coronary angioplasty with coronary bypass surgery: Emory Angioplasty versus Surgery Trial (EAST). *N Engl J Med* 331:1044-1050, 1994.

29. Hamm CW, Reimers J, Ischinger T, et al: A randomized study of coronary angioplasty compared with bypass surgery in patients with symptomatic multivessel coronary disease: German Angioplasty Bypass Surgery Investigation (GABI). *N Engl J Med* 331:1037-1043, 1994.

30. Rodriguez A, Boullon F, Perez-Balino N, et al: Argentine Randomized Trial of Percutaneous Transluminal Coronary Angioplasty Versus Coronary Artery Bypass Surgery in Multivessel Disease (ERACI): In-hospital results and 1-year follow-up. ERACI Group. *J Am Coll Cardiol* 22:1060-1067, 1993.

31. Williams DO, Baim DS, Bates E, et al: Coronary anatomic and procedural characteristics of patients randomized to coronary angioplasty in the Bypass Angioplasty Revascularization Investigation (BARI). *Am J Cardiol* 75:27C-33C, 1995.

32. Hlatky MA, Rogers WJ, Johnstone I, et al: Medical care costs and quality of life after randomization to coronary angioplasty or coronary bypass surgery. Bypass Angioplasty Revascularization Investigation (BARI) Investigators. *N Engl J Med* 336:92-99, 1997.

33. Pocock SJ, Henderson RA, Seed P, et al: Quality of life, employment status, and anginal symptoms after coronary angioplasty or bypass surgery. 3-Year follow-up in the Randomized Intervention Treatment of Angina (RITA) Trial. *Circulation* 94:135-142, 1996.

34. Sim I, Gupta M, McDonald K, et al: A meta-analysis of randomized trials comparing coronary artery bypass grafting with percutaneous transluminal coronary angioplasty in multivessel coronary artery disease. *Am J Cardiol* 76:1025-1029, 1995.

35. Jones RH, Kesler K, Phillips HR III, et al: Long-term survival benefits of coronary artery bypass grafting and percutaneous transluminal angioplasty in patients with coronary artery disease. *J Thorac Cardiovasc Surg* 111:1013-1025, 1996.

36. Puel J, Karouny E, Marco F, et al: Angioplasty versus surgery in multivessel disease: Immediate results and in-hospital outcomes in a randomized prospective study. *Circulation* 86:1-372, 1992.

37. Zhao XQ, Brown BG, Stewart DK, et al: Effectiveness of revascularization in the Emory Angioplasty versus Surgery Trial: A randomized comparison of coronary angioplasty with bypass surgery. *Circulation* 93:1954-1962, 1996.

38. Weintraub WS, Mauldin PD, Becker E, et al: A comparison of the costs of and quality of life after coronary angioplasty or coronary surgery for multivessel coronary artery disease: Results from the Emory Angioplasty versus Surgery Trial (EAST). *Circulation* 92:2831-2840, 1995.

39. Rodriguez A, Ahualli P, Perez-Balino N, et al: Argentine Randomized Trial of Percutaneous Transluminal Coronary Angioplasty versus Coronary Artery Bypass Surgery in Multivessel Disease (ERACI): Late cost and three years follow-up results. *J Am Coll Cardiol* 23:469A, 1994.

40. Randomized trials of PTCA: Comparison of medical and surgical therapy, in Grech ED, Ramdale DR (eds): *Practical Interventional Cardiology.* St Louis, Mosby, 1997, pp 317-326.

CHAPTER 2

Myocardial Revascularization Without Cardiopulmonary Bypass

Albert J. Pfister, M.D.

Assistant Clinical Professor in Surgery, The George Washington University School of Medicine; Senior Attending Surgeon, Washington Hospital Center, Washington, D.C.

Avoidance of cardiopulmonary bypass during myocardial revascularization has recently sparked much discussion by surgeons and cardiologists. This chapter will cover only coronary artery bypass without cardiopulmonary bypass grafting (off-pump CABG). Transmyocardial laser revascularization and gene therapy can also be done off pump, but those are beyond the scope of this chapter.

The topic of myocardial revascularization without cardiopulmonary bypass is a controversial one. It polarizes cardiac surgeons, with strong opinions expressed both pro and con. I am no exception. I feel that beating-heart CABG performed on properly selected patients is a good thing with tangible benefits. My opinions are scattered throughout this chapter; these are personal opinions and not gospel.

Much of this topic is concerned with technique. All the surgeons practicing at the Washington Hospital Center do beating-heart coronary surgery, and there is a free exchange of ideas and techniques. Clever little tricks and shortcuts abound to make the operations simpler, quicker, and safer. I will share some of these with you and will try to acknowledge their origin. Some have been around for so long that no one remembers who came up with them. I implore my colleagues to forgive me if I share one of their innovations without giving credit.

HISTORY

The original coronary artery bypasses were done without cardiopulmonary bypass.[1,2] However, in the mid-to-late 1960s, cardiopulmonary bypass technology became widespread and relatively safe. In addition, cardioplegic strategies became more practical. In fairly short order, direct coronary artery bypass done on pump with cardioplegic arrest became the gold standard for myocardial revascularization. The relative ease of performing microanastomoses in a motionless and bloodless field is obvious. More important than the ease of the operation was that cardiopulmonary bypass allowed the technique to be performed by almost all cardiac surgeons, with very reproducible results.

I must point out that I am a big fan of cardiopulmonary bypass. It is tremendous technology that allows us as cardiac surgeons to do wonderful things. It is not without a downside, however. The detrimental effects of bypass are well covered by excellent review articles.[3,4]

The initial attempts to revive off-pump CABG in the 1970s were met with less than an enthusiastic response.[5] In the 1980s, the large volume of pioneering work by Buffolo et al.[6] and Benetti et al.[7] in South America sparked a renewed interest in beating-heart coronary surgery. Much of that work was driven by economic concerns. The cost of cardiopulmonary bypass was prohibitive for many patients in those countries. The excellent results of Buffolo and Benetti encouraged our group in Washington, D.C., to begin performing beating-heart coronary surgery in the mid-1980s. I reported our results on 220 patients with matched controls at the 1990 Annual Meeting of the Society of Thoracic Surgeons.[8] I thought our report convincingly showed the safety and benefit of off-pump CABG. However, controversy remained.

The largest advance in beating-heart CABG, in my opinion, came in the early 1990s when mechanical stabilization for off-pump CABG was devised. Benetti,[9] working with a company called CardioThoracic Systems, produced a retractor and stabilizing system for the MIDCAB (Minimally Invasive Direct Coronary Artery Bypass, CardioThoracic Systems, Cupertino, CA) procedure. This was an operation designed originally to allow harvest of the left internal mammary artery (LIMA) under direct vision, and anastomosis of that LIMA to the left anterior descending (LAD) coronary artery off bypass through a small left anterior thoracotomy.[10]

We began performing MIDCABs at the Washington Hospital Center in June 1996, and we, like others were impressed that the mechanical stabilizer made the operation infinitely easier, and more important, more reproducible. It did not take long before we and others were using the MIDCAB retractor and stabilizer system to perform multivessel off-pump CABG via sternotomy. The instrument companies responded in fairly short order with a multitude of retractor and stabilizer systems designed for CABG via sternotomy and other incisions.

INDICATIONS

The indications for off-pump CABG can be either simple or complex, depending on the enthusiasm and experience of the surgeon. For zealots with a large experience, the answer is simple—the indication for beating-heart CABG is most, or even any, patient requiring coronary bypass.

For most surgeons, however, the answer is much more complex and must be individualized for each surgeon and patient. At my original presentation, I noted that our indications for off-pump surgery were clearly defined: (1) complete revascularization must be possible (this meant disease in the LAD and/or right coronary artery (RCA) systems only, because we initially considered the circumflex system to be unapproachable off pump), and (2) a reason exists to avoid cardiopulmonary bypass (e.g., redo, Jehovah's Witness, cerebrovascular disease, diseased ascending aorta). Specifically, I emphasized that the ability to perform the procedure is not an indication to do so.

For most surgeons, the decision to proceed with off-pump CABG will depend on two key issues: durability of their procedure and completeness of revascularization. The advantage of surgical revascularization over percutaneous techniques has always been complete revascularization with better long-term results.[11] These benchmarks must never be relinquished or compromised, though at times they can be bent if in the patient's best interest.

The first stumbling block is that optimal revascularization is not necessarily complete revascularization. One of my colleagues, Mercedes Dullum, is quick to point out that a live, optimally revascularized patient is better than a dead, completely revascularized one. This is common sense. A high-risk patient (old age, poor ventricular function, multiple comorbid conditions) may not need to have a small obtuse marginal grafted. Alternately, some coronary lesions are very amenable to percutaneous treatment, and it may be best for the patient to perform a hybrid procedure with part surgical, part percutaneous revascularization.[12] As procedures and techniques evolve and as experience grows, so do the options for each patient. A close and honest relationship between cardiologist and cardiac surgeon (at times a rarity) is necessary to keep the patient's best interests foremost.

Durability of the anastomosis is tantamount. The assessment regarding quality of anastomosis must be made by each surgeon during the procedure. Abandoning an anastomosis because of quality concerns should not be considered a failure but rather good judgment. Likewise, deciding in advance to perform CABG on pump because of quality of the target vessel or location of the lesion is commendable. The performance of marginal quality anastamoses (or as some put it, doing bypass with angioplasty backup) just so a procedure can be done off pump must be avoided.

My approach to indications for performing off-pump CABG is as follows. Assuming I feel all anastamoses can be done well, disease in the LAD and/or RCA systems by itself is an indication for off-pump CABG. The safety and benefits of that operation have been proven time and again by myself and others.[8,13,14] With regard to circumflex disease, I feel that the exposure and stabilization techniques are still variable from patient to patient and surgeon to surgeon. Consequently, before approaching a circumflex lesion off bypass, I feel that there must be a good reason to avoid cardiopulmonary bypass in the patient.

TECHNIQUES

Not to minimize the importance of clinical decision making, but the fact remains that the success or failure of off-pump CABG is mainly technical. I will discuss technical aspects of MIDCAB, multivessel CABG via sternotomy, and CABG via posterolateral thoracotomy.

There are a number of general considerations regarding off-pump CABG regardless of the incision. The first regards perfusion backup. When we began our beating-heart CABG experience, we not only had the perfusionist in the operating room, but also a pump set up and the lines handed onto the field. As we became more comfortable, we began eliminating these one by one. It is comforting to have a perfusionist in the operating room but not absolutely necessary, provided one is readily available. Pump status depends a lot on the nature of the case and the day's schedule. If the case is high risk or there is an on-pump case to follow in the operating room, I see no reason not to set up a wet pump (i.e., primed and ready to go). If the case is low risk and there is no case to follow, then a dry pump should suffice. I never do a case off bypass without perfusion being available. The question of the need for a cell saver is often raised. I do not feel that it is worthwhile for only one or two grafts. If I plan on doing more than that, the amount of blood retrieved likely will justify the cost of the apparatus.

I find a headlight almost a necessity. We do not use headlights routinely, but often the exposure is tedious and by necessity there are more hands in the field, which makes adequate lighting difficult. Likewise, we hardly ever use a second assistant, but with off-

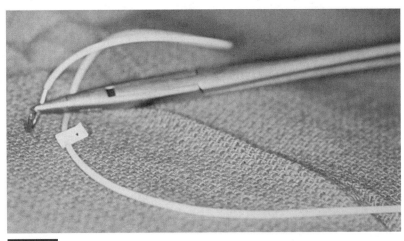

FIGURE 1.

The Silastic loop with blunt needle attached, used for proximal and/or distal control. Two holes are made in an ordinary pledget, using a 20-gauge needle. The Silastic loop is passed through one hole. The needle is then passed around the coronary artery and through the second hole. After opening the coronary artery, the pledget is snugged down to the epicardial surface and kept in place with a medium hemostatic clip, if necessary.

bypass cases, I feel one is necessary at least during the anastomosis. A second assistant is crucial mainly in keeping the anastomotic field clear of blood.

To help keep the field clear of blood, I use a carbon dioxide (CO_2) blower. With this technique I have found that distal control is almost never required. This, in turn, has eliminated the theoretical concern of stenosis at the snare site. Proximal control is by means of a Silastic loop bolstered with a pledget and held in place with a hemostatic clip, if needed (Fig 1). That technique I believe was devised by Rob Matheny and provides a relatively atraumatic and low-profile means of proximal control. If the target vessel is totally occluded, I don't even bother with proximal control. Our surgeons are split regarding shunts. All, however, make sure that one is available when working on the RCA.

I routinely give 10,000 units of heparin and monitor activated clotting times to keep them about 250 to 300 seconds. The surgeons at the Washington Hospital Center vary regarding their use of protamine after the completion of the anastomosis. I routinely give protamine. Postoperatively we use just an aspirin a day.

For MIDCABs and off-bypass CABG via posterolateral thoracotomy, I prefer to use a bronchial blocker to allow one lung ventilation, though this is not absolutely necessary. If the case has gone smoothly and the patient has no other risk factors preventing it, I prefer to attempt extubation in the operating room. For pain control, we use a variety of methods including intercostal blocks, patient-controlled analgesia pumps, epidural analgesia, and non-steroidal anti-inflammatory drugs. Temporary pacing wires are not routinely used. Cutaneous defibrillator pads (R2 patches) are routinely used for cases that are redo operations. Otherwise pediatric internal paddles are sufficient.

Most of the time I will perform proximal anastomoses before distals. It is important to keep the systolic pressure relatively low (about 90 mm Hg) during the period of partial occlusion to avoid clamp injury to the acsending aorta.

The importance of aggressive and attentive anesthesia and nursing cannot be stressed enough. With on-pump coronary surgery, the time of the distal anastomoses is often a "downtime" for anesthesia and nursing. The opposite is true for off-pump CABGs. When an instrument is needed, it usually is needed immediately. Hemodynamics can be variable depending on the amount of cardiac manipulation and displacement and temporary coronary occlusion. The success of off-pump CABG is truly dependent on a team effort.

Close study of the diagnostic angiogram usually will eliminate the situation of being surprised by an intramyocardial vessel. If encountered unexpectedly, an attempt can be made to expose the vessel. Using the electrocautery at a low level controls the venous bleeding from cut myocardium. Care must be taken to avoid fibrillating the heart. It is usually easier to expose such a vessel before applying the stabilizer. Alternatively, the procedure off pump can be abandoned and converted to on pump.

As previously mentioned, mechanical stabilizers have been the greatest technological improvement in beating-heart coronary surgery since its beginning. Some of these stabilizers are reusable, and some are disposable; some require a special retractor, and some attach to the retractors commonly available. All systems are relatively expensive. Consequently, the temptation is to eliminate them or to devise some homemade stabilization system. I feel that this is foolish. I have tried many homemade stabilizers, such as table forks with tines removed and endotracheal tube stylets bent and twisted in various configurations. To date, I believe I have also tried all the commercial stabilizers. In my opinion, there is no comparison. Granted, there is the occasional situation (especially with distal RCAs) where—after traction sutures have been placed and the heart positioned—the anastomotic site is stable enough that mechanical stabilization adds little. In the vast majority of cases and for the vast majority of surgeons, mechanical stabilization is crucial for the performance of a flawless anastomosis. I admit that the instruments can be expensive, but I submit that so is an angioplasty or a reoperation.

There are two basic types of stabilizers: traction or suction stabilizers (most notably the Octopus, Medtronic, Inc., Minneapolis, MN), and plate or compression stabilizers. It is important to keep in mind that the stabilizers are designed to do just that—stabilize the anastomotic site. To varying degrees, they can also aid in positioning the heart, but that should not be a major task.

The traction stabilizer (Octopus) is bulky and requires a significant learning curve to become comfortable using it. It seems to do a superior job in stabilizing the lateral vessels. I just recently had the opportunity to use the second-generation Octopus. It is much more compact and user-friendly than its predecessor. I am still experimenting with the Octopus and to date mainly use a plate stabilizer.

The design of compression stabilizers is similar from one manufacturer to the next. Almost all involve a foot or plate, attached to a post. Stabilization is best with these devices when the post is positioned at right angles (radially) to the anastomosis. The further the post is from 90 degrees, the less mechanical advantage it has and the more motion there will be.

The postoperative care of the off-pump CABG patient is basically the same as that of the patient done on pump. In general, though, the timetable for all landmarks (extubation, chest tube removal, first time out of bed) can be accelerated.

MIDCAB

I consider the MIDCAB to be a great operation for a very limited indication—that is, a single graft to an LAD. When we began doing MIDCABs at the Washington Hospital Center, we were very enthusiastic and as a consequence stretched the procedure. After numerous requests from the referring cardiologists to try two or more grafts via a small anterior thoracotomy (to the LAD, diagonals and/or ramus), we began to try sequential grafts. I feel that the results were less than satisfactory, and I now consider the MIDCABG to be strictly a single graft to LAD operation. Manny Subramanian has pointed out to me and others that the operation is ergonomically different than CABG via sternotomy. Even if you have been doing lots of off-pump coronary surgery via sternotomy, there is still a learning curve involved. By making the MIDCAB a single graft operation, it will represent a very small percentage of the typical surgeon's practice.

For almost all patients and almost all LAD lesions, an incision in the fourth intercostal space will be appropriate. Some individuals make a big deal about body habitus, lesion location, and shape of the heart. When I started performing MIDCABs, I would agonize over the chest x-ray, the catheterization films, and the patient. Then I would make the incision in the fourth intercostal space. Even if that incision does not put you exactly where you want to be, traction sutures and the stabilizer can help position things appropriately. Incision length varies with the size of the patient. The medial end should start about 5 cm lateral to the left sternal edge.

I think it is preferable to make the skin incision directly over the interspace desired. In men, this sometimes will be above the nipple, which is not a big deal. In woman, there are special considerations. I think that the skin incision in women needs to be at or near the inframammary fold. In some women, this is over the seventh or lower intercostal space. If the chest is to be entered at the fourth intercostal space, a lot of the breast must be elevated off the chest wall to get the exposure needed. Even then, especially in women with large breasts, the procedure can be difficult. Body habitus, in both men and women, can be a relative contraindication to MIDCAB.

After entry into the chest, the first thing to do is develop the potential space between the inside of the chest wall and the pericardial fat. That is why I say that the easiest first patient to perform a MIDCAB on is a thin, tall male with moderately severe chronic obstructive pulmonary disease. The space between the chest wall and the pericardium (which is the tunnel through which the LIMA is harvested) is spacious.

I expose the LIMA by incising the endothoracic fascia lateral to the lateral mammary vein, which almost always is right where the ribs turn to cartilage and start to curve back superiorly to meet the sternum. I then dissect from lateral to medial, or in a mirror-image fashion to the technique via sternotomy. Some individuals advocate coming down on the LIMA from above, but I find this cumbersome and more likely to damage the internal mamary artery (IMA).

In large patients, exposure can be difficult, and sometimes a Rultract (Rultract, Inc., Cleveland, OH) or other sternal retractor for IMA harvest via sternotomy can be hooked under the third rib to help increase that potential space between the chest wall and the pericardium. IMA harvest routinely goes from the sixth intercostal space to the subclavian vein. Superiorly, it is very important to divide the two or three medial pericardial vessels; otherwise, these will tether the IMA pedicle and shorten it.

I no longer agonize over the site for pericardiotomy. I just make a small (2-3 cm) vertical incision at a convenient location in the pericardium and then tailor it according to what I see. Pericardial traction sutures are crucial in presenting the anastomotic site into the operative field. The stabilizer can also be used to fine tune the vessel location.

After completion of the anastomosis, I use the usual two fine sutures to tack the IMA pedicle to the epicardium. In addition, I use a third to tack the pedicle to the apex of the pericardiotomy. This prevents displacement of the pedicle by the lung when the left lung is ventilated again. Before making the pericardiotomy, I raise a flap of pericardial fat that I save and then place over the anastomosis to protect it, should a reoperation via sternotomy ever be required.

I routinely use intercostal blocks before closing. I use a small chest tube for drainage, although some use a small suction drain. Either are adequate.

If the IMA is injured or is found to be unusable, the operation does not necessarily have to be abandoned and converted to a sternotomy. If another conduit is available (saphenous vein graft, radial artery, short piece of free IMA), a proximal anastomosis can be performed to the ascending aorta through the small anterior thoracotomy incision. Traction sutures are put in the pericardium anterior to the superior vena cava, and using these, the ascending aorta is presented so that a small partial occlusion clamp can be applied.

OFF-BYPASS CABG VIA STERNOTOMY

When we began doing MIDCABs, it was not long before we began using the stabilizer platform to perform multivessel CABG off bypass using a sternotomy incision. There are now a number of retractor and stabilizer systems available specifically for this indication. The main points to be made in this section regard order of anastomosis and exposure of the three main coronary systems.

Intuitively, one would think that the most logical order of anastomoses would be from least ischemic vessel to most ischemic; or is it from most ischemic to least ischemic? In my opinion, it doesn't really matter. More important is that anastomoses be done in the order of least amount of cardiac displacement to most. In other words, do the anastomosis that will result in the least amount of hemodynamic disruption first. For most patients, this means that the order of anastomoses will be the LAD/diagonal system, followed by the RCA/posterior descending coronary artery (PDA) system, followed by the circumflex system.

The question is often asked—if I've never done any beating-heart coronary surgery before but am interested in starting, what should be my first anastomosis? The answer is easy: an LAD via sternotomy. The anastomosis is familiar, comfortable, stable, and remarkably well tolerated. To set up such an anastomosis, pericardial traction sutures are used to stabilize the left half of the pericardial well. Then the

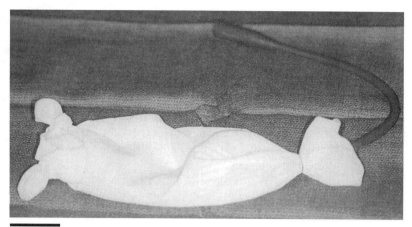

FIGURE 2.
"The glove."

heart needs to be displaced anterior and to the right to present the LAD. Up until about 6 months ago, I used to use a number of warm lap pads to do that job. My friend, Mercedes Dullum, helped devise "the glove" (Fig 2)—a red rubber catheter tied into an ordinary sterile glove (I tie off the fingers because they look funny when the glove is inflated) that is then placed underneath the heart in the pericardial well. The end of the red rubber catheter is left out and is used to inflate the glove with warm saline. The nicest thing about this system is that it allows very gradual displacement of the heart. Gradual displacement translates into gradual hemodynamic changes, which makes this system very endearing to the anesthesiologists. It allows the individuals at the head of the table to compensate for any dip in blood pressure. If the displacement is too great, a syringe-full of saline can be withdrawn to allow anesthesia to catch up and then be reinstilled when the numbers have improved. The glove has made LAD/diagonal sequential grafts fairly routine. The heart is slowly displaced to allow performance of the diagonal anastomosis, then some saline can be withdrawn for the LAD anastomosis (Figs 3 and 4).

There are a variety of ways to approach the RCA/PDA system. I will describe what works for me. First, the patient is placed in a steep Trendelenberg positon. Then two traction sutures are placed through the acute margin of the right ventricle. It is usually best to use pledgeted monofilament material. The first is placed at the junction of the acute margin with the right atrium, very near the course of the right coronary artery. This suture is then attached to the drapes toward the patient's right shoulder. The second stitch is put through the acute margin about halfway to the apex. It is attached to the drapes toward the left shoulder of the patient (Fig 5). Some ten-

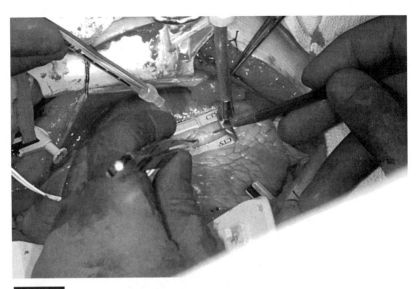

FIGURE 3.

Exposing the left anterior descending coronary artery. Note pericardial traction sutures in place; the glove at the inferior portion of the sternotomy; the left internal mammary artery, which had been previously prepared, on the *left side* of the picture; the CO_2 blower in place, being held by the second assistant; and the fact that the post on the stabilizer apparatus approaches the heart in a radial fashion for maximum stabilization.

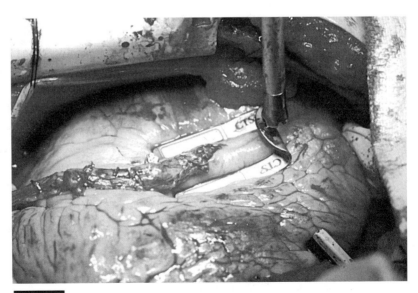

FIGURE 4.

Completed left internal mammary artery to left anterior descending coronary artery anastomosis. The Silastic loop for proximal control can be seen just before removal.

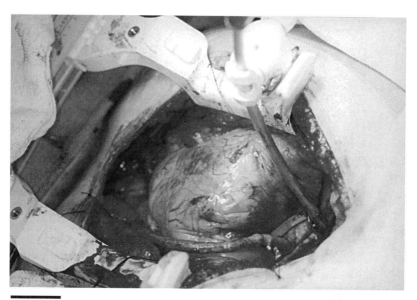

FIGURE 5.
Completed saphenous vein graft to posterior descending branch of the right coronary artery. Notice that the patient is in steep Trendelenberg position, and the two traction sutures as described in the text, pulling the acute margin of the heart superiorly.

sion can be taken off these stitches by bolstering the diaphragmatic surface of the heart with warm lap pads or with "the glove."

The right coronary system is the most sensitive to ischemia. Consequently, it can be the most terrifying system to deal with off bypass. I am constantly amazed at how sick a patient can get with occlusion of a right coronary artery. Because of this, I always try to do my distal anastomosis to the PDA rather than the RCA. In addition, I always have a shunt in the room when doing RCA work.

I have always said that I have never abandoned an anastomosis because of ischemia. That was true until about 2 months ago. I was operating on a patient with critical LAD, diagonal, and RCA disease. She had recently been admitted with an inferior infarct. In keeping with the strategy as outlined above, I proceeded with the diagonal anastomosis first. While positioning the heart for that anastomosis, I got a little bit ahead of anesthesia and the systolic pressure dropped to about 80 mm Hg. The patient became acutely ischemic in the RCA distribution with inferior ST elevation. This was refractory to all medical management, and I had to convert the patient to on bypass.

Clearly, the circumflex system is the most difficult to approach off bypass via sternotomy. It is relatively easy through a thoracotomy (see below).

In certain patients, it is not possible to do the circumflex off bypass, no matter how many maneuvers are done. The large heart with poor function usually will not tolerate the manipulation required for exposure. In general, regardless of what technique is used to present the target vessel, the anastomosis will be further distal on the coronary artery than if the procedure was done on bypass.

I recommend that the circumflex system be attempted only after the surgeon has gained a substantial experience with off-bypass work on the LAD and RCA systems. The plan of attack needs to be very focused and organized. Repeated positioning or prolonged manipulation is usually not tolerated. Hesitation is counterproductive. Unlike the LAD system where, for the most part, almost unlimited time is available to do the anastomosis, such is not the case with obtuse marginals. That sense of urgency needs to be shared by everyone in the operating room.

There are two main techniques that are used to expose the obtuse marginals. Both techniques rely on gravity to help with positioning, so the patient is placed in a steep Trendelenberg position and the table is rolled to the right. Antonio Calafiore uses a system of slings made of vaginal packing. Two slings are brought

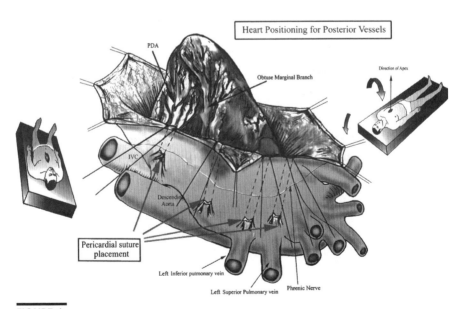

FIGURE 6.
Depiction of one technique to expose the lateral and posterior vessels. Notice traction sutures deep in the pericardial well, just anterior to the pulmonary veins, and the fact that the patient is in steep Trendelenberg and rotated to his right. *Abbreviations: PDA,* posterior descending coronary artery; *IVC,* inferior vena cava. (Courtesy of CardioThoracic Systems, Inc.)

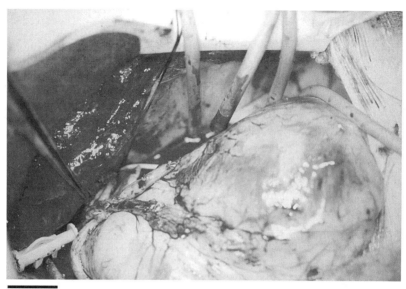

FIGURE 7.

Just before making the arteriotomy for a graft to the obtuse marginal. Previous left internal mammary artery to left anterior descending coronary artery, and saphenous vein graft to diagonal branch are visible on the *left side* of the photograph. Traction sutures can be seen. The inferior traction sutures have been covered wtih red rubber catheters to prevent them from abrading the epicardial surface of the heart. The stabilizer is in place, approaching the heart from the patient's left side.

through the transverse sinus, and two are brought behind the inferior vena cava. This leaves four ends on each side of the heart. The free ends on the left side of the heart are crossed to bracket the target vessel and brought over to the right side and fixed to the drapes. This elevates the heart out of the chest and brings it to a near vertical position. Volume loading and liberal use of a pressor are often needed to maintain acceptable hemodynamics.

The other technique, and the one that I prefer, was developed by Lima in South America and has been championed by Salerno and others in the United States. It involves a series of pericardial traction sutures placed very low on the left side, just anterior to the pulmonary veins. These are then fixed to the drapes on the patient's left side. Again, the heart is displaced out of the chest and made vertical, with the apex pointing toward the ceiling (Fig 6).

With either technique the compression stabilizer usually works best if brought in from the patient's left side (Figs 7 and 8).

Suction stabilizers usually work best if brought in from the right side and reach over the heart. Most of the positioning should be done with sutures, slings, and bolsters and not with the stabilizer.

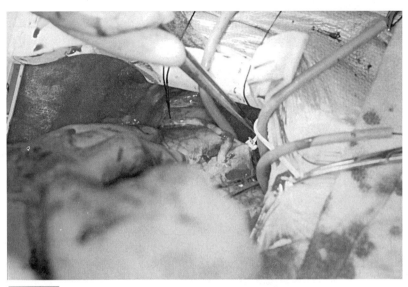

FIGURE 8.
Completed saphenous vein graft to obtuse marginal coronary artery. Notice traction sutures in place and Silastic loop for proximal control.

CABG OFF PUMP VIA POSTEROLATERAL THORACOTOMY

For years, the standard coronary bypass operation involved a LIMA grafted to the LAD with saphenous vein grafts for all other vessels. Our practice at the Washington Hospital Center, as at other centers, is to perform not only a higher percentage of redo coronary operations but also a higher percentage of redo operations with a patent IMA graft. Typically, the LIMA is not only patent, but also crucial, often being the only functioning graft. In addition, 10 or more years ago, not many surgeons were thinking about reoperations when using IMA grafts. Consequently, those grafts are frequently in precarious positions with regards to a repeat sternotomy.

If the patient only requires regrafting of the circumflex system, there is another approach that permits the case to be done off bypass and also avoids risk to the patent LIMA. A left posterolateral thoracotomy gives excellent exposure to the obtuse marginals.

Conduit, whether it be saphenous vein or radial artery, needs to be harvested before positioning the patient in the lateral decubitus position. As with MIDCABs, a bronchial blocker that allows single lung ventilation is helpful, though not a requirement. I enter the chest through the fifth intercostal space. Any adhesions to the lower lobe and lingula are lysed and the inferior pulmonary ligament is divided, so the lung can be retracted superiorly. The pericardium is opened posterior to the phrenic nerve. Usually the old graft can be used as a guide to the target vessel. The proximal anastomosis can be placed in a variety of locations. Most convenient, and requiring the least length of conduit, is the descending thoracic aorta. If this site is chosen, keep in mind that when the lung reexpands, it will push the graft inferiorly. Alternately, the subclavian or even the axillary artery can be used for inflow.

RESULTS

Our group operates out of three area hospitals: The Washington Hospital Center in Washington, D.C., The Washington Adventist Hospital in Takoma Park, Maryland, and Union Memorial Hospital in Baltimore, Maryland. The following results represent those of all the surgeons in our group at the two Maryland hospitals, and all the surgeons at the Washington Hospital Center.

From June 15, 1996 through November 1998, we performed MID-CAB on 265 patients, which represents 275 grafts. There were two deaths in this group for an overall mortality rate of 0.8%.

From January 1, 1985 through November 1998, a total of 1,012 patients had CABG done off bypass, representing a total of 1,401 grafts. Of this cohort of 1,012 patients, 265 had a MIDCAB, 24 had their coronary bypass via a posterolateral thoracotomy, and 723 patients had CABG off pump via a sternotomy. This group of 723 patients represents 1,098 grafts. Mortality data are sketchy for the group from 1985 to 1990, with close to 70 patients lost to follow-up in our database. The group from 1990 through November 1998 had an overall mortality rate of 2.2%.

Other than the recent Patency Outcome and Economics of MID-CAB (POEM) trial patients, the most closely scrutinized group has been those patients (all redos) who have had their CABG off bypass via a left posterolateral thoracotomy. From January 1, 1996 through November 1998, we have operated on 24 such patients, representing 28 grafts. We have complete follow-up on the first 19 of those patients. There were no deaths. Eighteen of 19 patients required no further intervention, and 17 of those 19 are angina-free.

MYTHS

The topic of myocardial revascularization without cardiopulmonary bypass is a controversial one. At times, emotion precludes reason. Let me present, and hopefully dispel, a number of myths regarding beating-heart coronary surgery that I frequently encounter.

1. "My patency for a LIMA to LAD done on bypass is 100%. The patency for that anastomosis done off bypass is much worse."
   This is more a statement of ignorance than of fact. The truth is that very few surgeons know what their graft patency rate is

because few asymptomatic patients have follow-up catheterizations performed. Pioneering work by Calafiore[15] has shown that the perfect patency rate for a LIMA to LAD done on bypass is between 92% and 95%. A recent thoughtful review by Mack et al.[16] exposed the problems with trying to arrive at a patency number for that graft. I do know that with the POEM trial, our LIMA to LAD anastomoses have become the most closely scrutinized grafts, with angiography performed on postoperative day 2 or 3 and at 6 months. To date, 20 such patients have had their 72-hour postoperative angiogram. Nineteen of those grafts have been patent. Nine patients thus far have returned for their 6-month postoperative angiogram. The patency of these grafts is 100%.

2. "The retractor and stabilizer systems for the most part are disposable and expensive. They increase the cost of a routine CABG."

   You will get no argument from me regarding the cost of the instrumentation. However, with elimination of pump costs and with fewer days in the hospital, we have repeatedly found that the total cost of CABG done off bypass is about 20% less than on bypass.

3. "I like to do CABGs off pump because it's faster."

   This is true and false. A single graft done off pump is, in general, quicker than doing the same graft on pump. However, when multiple grafts are done off pump, those operations tend to be longer than their on-pump counterparts. Positioning of the heart and stabilizing the anastomosis and hemodynamics take a significant amount of time. In addition, it often takes the heart 10 or 15 minutes between anastomoses to recover from the manipulation. Finally, the entire extubation ritual adds significantly to operating room time.

4. "I do so much of my coronary work off pump that I'm thinking of laying off my perfusionists."

   With rare exception, beating-heart coronary surgery will represent much less than 50% of a surgeon's practice. Also, I can't imagine doing an off-pump case without perfusion backup.

CONCLUSIONS

At a recent social gathering for local cardiac surgeons, I was a bit surprised when an informal poll showed that 50% would still want to have their LIMA to LAD done on bypass with aortic cross clamping and cardioplegic arrest. All of those who chose to have their graft done off pump made the point that they would pick their surgeon and hospital very carefully.

There are many potential benefits to be derived from off-pump coronary bypass. These include shorter ICU and hospital stays, shorter time to extubation, lower incidence of transfusion, and lower incidence of the need for inotropic support with or without intra-aortic balloon pump. In addition, high-risk patients—those who are older, have severely impaired ventricular function, or have multiple comorbid conditions—do significantly better if their CABG can be done off pump.[8,17,18] Still, the procedure is not for all surgeons, nor for all patients. The learning curve can be substantial, and with unbridled enthusiasm, the results can be suboptimal. New techniques and instrumentation are being developed at an intoxicating rate, often surrounded with a healthy dose of public relation hype. I feel it mandatory to maintain a cautious, but open frame of mind during this very exciting time in cardiac surgery.

REFERENCES

1. Murray G, Porcheron R, Hilano J, et al: Anastomosis of a systemic artery to the coronary. *Can Med Assoc J* 71:594-597, 1954.
2. Kolesov V: Mammary artery–coronary artery anastomosis as a method for treating angina pectoris. *J Thorac Cardiovasc Surg* 54:535-544, 1967.
3. Butler J, Rocker GM, Westaby S: Inflammatory response to cardiopulmonary bypass. *Ann Thorac Surg* 55:552-559, 1993.
4. Edmunds LH: Why cardiopulmonary bypass makes patients sick: Strategies to control the blood-synthetic surface interface, in Karp RB, Laks H, Wechsler AS (eds): *Advances in Cardiac Surgery*, vol 6. St Louis, Mosby, 1995, pp 131-167.
5. Trapp WG, Bisarya R: Placement of coronary artery bypass graft without pump oxygenator. *Ann Thorac Surg* 19:108-109, 1975.
6. Buffolo E, Andrade JCS, Branco JNR, et al: Myocardial revascularization without extra-corporeal circulation: Seven year experience in 593 cases. *Eur J Cardiothorac Surg* 4:504-508, 1990.
7. Benetti FJ, Naselli G, Wood M, et al: Direct myocardial revascularization without extracorporeal circulation: Experience in 700 patients. *Chest* 100:312-316, 1991.
8. Pfister AJ, Zaki MS, Garcia JM, et al: Coronary artery bypass without cardiopulmonary bypass. *Ann Thorac Surg* 54:1085-1091, 1992.
9. Subramanian VA, Sani G, Benetti FJ, et al: Minimally invasive coronary bypass surgery: A multi-center report of preliminary clinical experience (abstract). *Circulation* 92(suppl I):1-645, 1995.
10. Calafiore AM, Di Gianmarco G, Teodori G, et al: Left anterior descending coronary artery grafting via left anterior small thoracotomy without cardiopulmonary bypass. *Ann Thorac Surg* 61:1658-1665, 1996.
11. Comparison of coronary bypass surgery with angioplasty in patients with multivessel disease. The Bypass Angioplasty Revascularization Investigation (BARI) Investigators. *N Engl J Med* 335:217-225, 1996.
12. Angelini GD, Wilde P, Salerno TA, et al: Integrated left small thoracotomy and angioplasty for multi-vessel coronary artery revascularisation. *Lancet* 347:757-758, 1996.

13. Buffolo E, de Andrade CS, Branco JN, et al: Coronary artery bypass grafting without cardiopulmonary bypass. *Ann Thorac Surg* 61:10-11, 1996.

14. Moshkovitz Y, Lusky A, Mohr R: Coronary artery bypass without cardiopulmonary bypass: Analysis of short-term and mid-term outcome in 220 patients. *J Thorac Cardiovasc Surg* 110:979-987, 1995.

15. Calafiore AM: Off pump coronary artery bypass. Surgical Grand Rounds, Washington Hospital Center, Washington, DC, October 1997.

16. Mack MJ, Osborne JA, Shennib H: Arterial graft patency in coronary artery bypass grafting: What do we really know? *Ann Thorac Surg* 66:1055-1059, 1998.

17. Magovern JA, Benckart DH, Landreneau RJ, et al: Morbidity, cost, and six-month outcome of minimally invasive direct coronary artery bypass grafting. *Ann Thorac Surg* 66:1224-1229, 1998.

18. Del Rizzo DF, Boyd WD, Novich RJ, et al: Safety and cost-effectiveness of MIDCABG in high-risk CABG patients. *Ann Thor Surg* 66:1002-1007, 1998.

CHAPTER 3

Transmyocardial Laser Revascularization

K.M. Cherian, M.S., F.R.A.C.S.
Professor Emeritus, M.G.R. Medical University; Director and Chief of
Cardiac Surgery, Institute of Cardiovascular Diseases, Madras, India

Ravi Agarwal, M.S., M.Ch.
Staff Surgeon, Institute of Cardiovascular Diseases, Madras, India

N. Madhu Sankar, M.S., Ph.D., D.N.B.
Consultant Cardiac Surgeon, Institute of Cardiovascular Diseases,
Madras, India

After the routine acceptance of coronary artery bypass grafting (CABG) and percutaneous coronary angioplasty (PTCA) procedures, various advances have been made to improve the results, such as total arterial revascularization in CABG and use of stents after PTCA. However, their use is limited to patients with good distal vessels and discrete lesions. In patients with diffuse coronary artery disease, the results of CABG have been suboptimal despite ancillary procedures such as endarterectomy, and little progress has been made to improve the results in this group of patients. Thus, there remains a subset of patients with diffusely diseased small-caliber vessels, having disabling angina despite maximal medical therapy who are not amenable to traditional methods of revascularization. Transmyocardial laser revascularization (TMLR) is a unique intervention that involves the creation of transmural channels in ischemic myocardium.[1] There is emerging evidence of the efficacy of TMLR in relieving anginal symptoms and improving myocardial perfusion in patients with diffuse coronary artery disease.

HISTORICAL PERSPECTIVE

Since the beginning of this century, various techniques of direct revascularization of the ischemic myocardium have been explored by many workers. Beck[2] proposed omentopexy and mypopexy in 1935 to induce capillary formation and to take advantage of neoangiogenesis in the myocardium. Intramyocardial implantation of the internal mammary artery by Vineberg[3] in 1946 was another step in this direction, and patent arteriomyocardial connections have been noted even after two decades. Further efforts were made to place conduits between myocardial sinusoids and the left ventricular cavity. Implantation of T tubes with the "leg of T" extending into the left ventricular cavity had been reported by Massimo and Baffi.[4] Sen et al.[5] studied the possibility of transventricular needle puncture to revascularize the ischemic myocardium. In 1970, Walter et al.[6] from Germany systematically investigated these procedures in a model of acute ischemia. However, rapid clotting of channels, prevented long-term success with these methods. In 1988, Mirhoseini et al.[1] introduced the carbon dioxide (CO_2) laser for TMLR, because its wavelength in the infrared range (10.6 nm) favors high absorption by biological tissue, thus permitting rapid tissue vaporization with minimal thermal damage to surrounding tissue. Clinical studies involving the use of TMLR started in 1990, and by now more than 2,000 procedures have been performed globally.

SELECTION OF PATIENTS

Patients with angina refractory to maximal medical therapy and coronary anatomy unsuitable for traditional methods of revascularization are selected for isolated TMLR. Patients with at least one graftable vessel are offered a combined procedure, even if the vessel is diffusely diseased and an endarterectomy is required. Patients with severe left ventricular dysfunction have been found to be unsuitable for isolated TMLR, and they are offered TMLR only as an adjunct procedure if they have at least one vessel suitable for bypass grafting. Patients with left ventricular aneurysms, bleeding diatheses, and morbid ventricular arrhythmias are considered unsuitable for TMLR.

PREOPERATIVE EVALUATION

The assessment of patients selected for TMLR is similar to that for patients undergoing CABG and includes routine biochemical and hematologic profiles, a 12-lead ECG, exercise stress testing, 2-dimensional echocardiography, and coronary angiography. Coagulation parameters are studied in detail to rule out the risk of major bleeding. The preoperative stress testing and echocardiographic analysis are standardized to provide a baseline against which the postoperative results will be compared. Thallium scintigraphic studies are performed to locate the areas of viable but ischemic myocardium, which is helpful in mapping the areas of myocardium to be lased. These studies are useful in assessing the improvement in myocardial perfusion during the follow-up period. The decision to perform TMLR as an isolated procedure or as an adjunct to CABG is based on the graftability of vessels as seen on coronary angiography.

ANESTHETIC MANAGEMENT

Prominent signboards indicating the use of a laser are displayed in the operating room, and protective eyewear is used by operating room personnel. The patients are prone to acute ischemic events, and all precautions for management of these should be undertaken. The full range of hemodynamic monitoring devices, including invasive arterial pressure monitoring, a pulmonary artery catheter, and transesophageal echocardiography, are used. Transesophageal echocardiography is useful in assessing ventricular contractility and regional wall motion abnormalities, and in confirming transmural penetration of channels. The ECG leads are connected to the patient as well as to the TMLR console. In patients undergoing isolated TMLR through a lateral thoracotomy, thoracic epidural analgesia is useful in controlling postoperative pain and allows early extubation. In patients undergoing combined TMLR and CABG, only partial postbypass reversal of heparin may be helpful in preserving the patency of channels as well as enhancing the flow through the grafts to small-caliber target coronary arteries.

SURGICAL TECHNIQUE
ISOLATED TMLR

A left anterolateral thoracotomy is performed through the fifth left intercostal space. The left lung is deflated, the pericardium is opened anterior to the phrenic nerve, and pericardial stay sutures are applied. The areas of ischemic myocardium to be lased are identified, avoiding areas with plentiful epicardial fat and scar tissue. An 800-W CO_2 laser (The Heart Laser, PLC Medical Inc., Milford, Mass) is used to create the laser channels using an energy output of 40 J and a pulse duration of 50 msec. Lately we have reduced the pulse duration to 25 msec because an experimental study has shown that the longer the pulse duration, the higher the risk of thermal damage to the surrounding tissues.[7] The laser is synchronized to the ECG signal and fired at the peak of the R wave. The laser energy is absorbed by blood in the ventricle. Transmyocardial penetration of laser is confirmed by a gush of

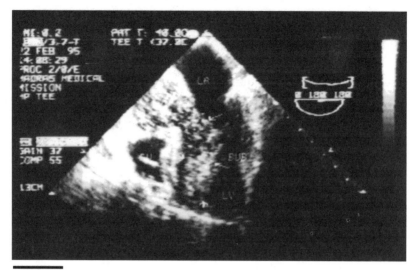

FIGURE 1.
Intraoperative transesophageal echocardiogram showing the bubbles (*BUB*) inside the left ventricle (*LV*). *Abbreviations: LA,* left atrium; *RV,* right ventricle.

bright red blood from the channel and detection of bubbles on transesophageal echocardiography (Fig 1). Bleeding from the channels is controlled by digital pressure and use of fresh blood coagulum. Usually 10 to 40 channels are created over different areas of ventricle with approximately 1-cm distance between the holes. After hemostasis, the pericardium is loosely approximated, and the wound is closed in layers with a drain.

COMBINED TMLR AND CABG

The procedure is performed through a median sternotomy on standard cardiopulmonary bypass. The graftable vessels are bypassed in the usual manner on fibrillatory arrest and intermittent cross clamping. The areas of viable myocardium not supplied by a graftable vessel are selected for TMLR. The patient is rewarmed to 34°C, and the perfusionist is asked to fill up the heart and allow it to eject. The laser channels are created at this stage using the same setting as for isolated TMLR. After completion of the procedure, the heart is decompressed again and allowed to recover on full bypass for 15 to 20 minutes, and only then is cardiopulmonary bypass terminated in the routine manner.

COMBINED TMLR AND CABG WITH ENDARTERECTOMY

Endarterectomy is performed if the vessel is completely occluded by atheromatous plaque, or the walls are calcareous preventing accurate suture placement. The right coronary artery is dealt with first and endarterectomy, if required, is done on fibrillatory arrest, followed by insertion of an onlay patch using saphenous vein. The proximal anastomosis is performed after release of the aortic clamp, on the empty beating heart. The left circumflex branches and the left anterior descending (LAD) artery are dealt with in a similar manner. After completion of grafting, TMLR is performed.

OUR EXPERIENCE

From December 1994 to November 1998, 193 patients underwent TMLR in our institution using a high-energy CO_2 laser. There were 182 men and 11 women, and their ages ranged from 39 to 76 years (mean age, 54.4 years). Sixty-seven patients (40.4%) had systemic hypertension and 81 (48.8%) were diabetic.

The patients were divided into four groups according to the type of procedure performed.

GROUP 1: ISOLATED TMLR (n = 108)

Patients in group 1 underwent TMLR as the sole procedure through a small left anterolateral thoracotomy. Their mean age (± SD) was 56.2 ± 9.2 years and 92.15% were men. Their mean preoperative angina class and ejection fraction were 2.6 ± 0.7 and 44.7% ± 10.5%, respectively. Diabetes mellitus was present in 49.01% of the patients, 32.3% had a history of previous myocardial infarction, and 12.7% had undergone previous CABG. The average number of holes created in each patient was 23 ± 8. Most of the patients were extubated within 8 to 12 hours after surgery. The mean duration of ventilation was 10.2 ± 4.4 hours, and the patients stayed in the ICU for a mean period of 2.6 ± 1.2 days. They were discharged on postoperative day 9, on average. An intra-aortic balloon pump was used in 11 patients because of low cardiac output, persistent myocardial ischemia, an evolving myocardial infarct, or an increasing need for inotropic support. Only 3 patients survived in this group, and the other 8 died of cardiac failure. Seventeen patients (15.7%) died in the hospital.

Univariate analysis of the predictors of early mortality revealed that female sex, advanced age, and perioperative myocardial infarction were factors significantly affecting the early mortality. The mean age of the patients who died was 63.1 years as compared with 56.6 years for those who survived the surgery. Other variables such as preoperative angina class, associated risk factors, previous myocardial infarction, and number of laser channels were not found to be predictors of early mortality. A multivariate logistic regression analysis was performed, and only age greater than 55 years was found to be a statistically significant predictor of early mortality (odds ratio, 7.7; 95% confidence interval, 16-36.7; $P < 0.01$).

Two patients died during follow-up; one died of myocardial infarction and the other died of sudden cardiac arrest. Other patients are seen regularly for follow-up, and their improvement in anginal status has continued at 1 year. The exercise capacity on treadmill both in exercise duration and metabolic equivalent load, which did not show any significant change up to 6 months after surgery, improved remarkably and gained statistical significance at 1-year follow-up. Thallium myocardial perfusion scans performed before surgery and 3 months after surgery did not reveal any significant improvement in myocardial perfusion.

GROUP 2: TMLR COMBINED WITH CABG (n = 41)
There were 37 men and 4 women in group 2, and their ages ranged from 38 to 68 years (mean age ± SD, 54.2 ± 7.6 years). Eighteen patients (43.9%) were hypertensive and 19 (46.3%) were diabetic. Eighteen patients had a history of previous myocardial infarction, and 4 had undergone previous CABG. The mean preoperative angina class was 2.5 ± 0.6, and 38% had unstable angina. The average number of grafts was 2.6 (range, 1-4), and the average number of holes was 12 ± 6. There were 5 hospital deaths; 2 were caused by low cardiac output and 3 resulted from perioperative myocardial infarction. The remaining patients are being followed up regularly over a period of 1 to 28 months. A reduction in antianginal medications has been reported by 60.5% of patients; 66% of patients are in angina class 1 or 2, and 15% continue to be in class 3. During follow-up, 1 patient died of ventricular arrhythmias.

GROUP 3: TMLR COMBINED WITH CABG AND ENDARTERECTOMY (n = 44)
There were 41 men and 3 women in group 3, and their ages ranged from 36 to 69 years (mean age ± SD, 53.7 ± 8.3 years). Twenty-one patients had a history of previous myocardial infarction, and 13 patients had unstable angina. Eighteen patients needed multiple endarterectomies. Twenty-four patients required endarterectomy of the LAD artery, and the left internal mammary artery was used as an onlay patch in 5 of these patients. The number of grafts ranged from 1 to 4, with an average of 2.85 per patient. The number of channels ranged from 8 to 24, with a mean of 10.8 ± 4 holes per patient. Five patients required an intra-aortic balloon pump in the perioperative period.

During the early postoperative period, a majority of patients in this group showed an increase in cardiac enzyme levels, ranging from 50 to 2,160 U/L of creatine kinase (mean, 478.4 U/L), 1% to 9% of the MB fraction of creatine kinase (mean, 3.94%), and 98 to 539 U/L of lactate dehydrogenase (mean, 259.4 U/L). Four patients

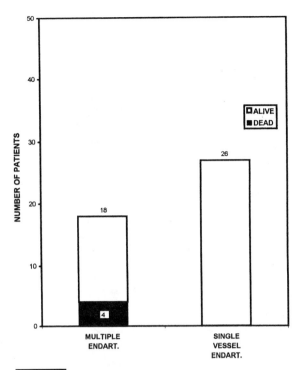

FIGURE 2.
Multiple-vessel endarterectomy and mortality.

died in the hospital; two patients died of intractable ventricular arrhythmias, and two died of low cardiac output. Analysis of our results showed that the risk of in-hospital mortality is significantly higher in patients requiring multiple-vessel endarterectomy compared with those who need single-vessel endarterectomy (Fig 2). Endarterectomy involving the LAD artery was found to be associated with higher in-hospital mortality compared with non-LAD endarterectomy, even though it was not significant statistically (Fig 3). The higher mortality in these patients may be attributed to use of the internal mammary artery. Thirty-three patients (86.8%) showed freedom from angina at 6 months. Four patients had angina on exertion and exhibited class 2 symptoms. One patient who had unstable angina preoperatively has shown no improvement and has been hospitalized for the angina.

GROUP 4: TMLR AND ASSOCIATED PROCEDURES (n = 2)

One patient underwent TMLR and closure of the sinus venosus type of atrial septal defect. The other patient underwent TMLR and a left upper lobectomy. For study purposes, these two patients were included in the isolated TMLR group (group 1).

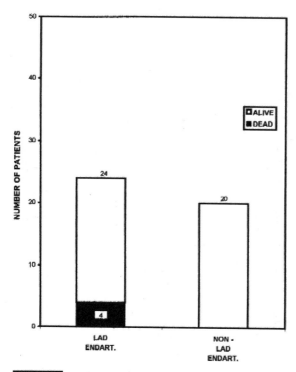

FIGURE 3.
Left anterior descending (*LAD*) endarterectomy (*ENDART.*) and mortality.

HISTOPATHOLOGY

Detailed histopathologic analysis was performed on the hearts of 11 patients who died in the hospital. The study of serial sections revealed that the epicardial end of the channel appeared depressed and filled with fibrin. The interesting feature observed was that none of the channels were found to be in a straight line. Rather they were twisted and taking a spiral course. Unless care is taken to cut large sections through and through, following the channels, it is likely to miss the course and conclude that the channel was closed. The apparent twisting of the channels is presumably caused by the architecture of the cardiac muscle and the contractility of myocardium at the time of creation of the channels. The majority of the channels were filled with plasma and erythrocytes separated by fibrin strands. The channels were found to be communicating with sinusoids in a large number of areas or opening into the endocardium, The endocardial area did show a few fibrin strands but they appeared to be of recent origin, indicating patency during life.

DISCUSSION

TMLR is a unique and modern therapeutic approach in the management of patients with diffuse coronary artery disease. Clinical data from various centers regularly performing TMLR are available now, and all of them consistently show a definite symptomatic improvement in angina class.[8-11] In many cases, the doses of antianginal medications could be reduced to less than 50% of the preoperative doses, and the average number of hospital admissions decreased from 2.5 ± 2 per year to 0.4 ± 0.6 per year. Further analysis of follow-up studies showed a definite improvement in exercise tolerance, and the benefit is sustained over a period of time (Table 1). However, there is no significant improvement in the ejection fraction. Multicenter trials from the United States with an experience of 200 patients have concluded that TMLR provides relief from anginal symptoms in patients with vessels unsuitable for other revascularization procedures. Furthermore, using the interventricular septum as a control, they have objectively demonstrated increased perfusion in the laser-treated left ventricular free wall, and these improvements were most apparent between 3 and 6 months and have persisted after 1 and 2 years. Cooley et al.[12,13] performed positron emission tomography scans before and after TMLR to study the differences in subepicardial and subendocardial perfusion, and they have demonstrated significant improvement in subendocardial perfusion after TMLR. Contrary to the popular belief that TMLR is not advisable in patients with left ventricular dysfunction, Lutter et al.[14] have reported seven cases of sole TMLR performed in patients with poor left ventricular function supported by a preoperatively inserted intra-aortic balloon pump. Encouraged by their good results, they have postulated that preoperative insertion of a balloon pump provides cardiac support during the postoperative phase of reversible decline of left ventricular function induced by TMLR.

Compared with the general Western population, our patients are much younger (mean age ± SD, 56.7 ± 9.2 years), with a greater number having diabetes (42%) and diffusely diseased small-caliber vessels. The major criticism of TMLR is its high early mortality, which has been attributed to perioperative myocardial infarction leading to cardiac failure. Although some degree of increase in cardiac enzyme levels has been noticed in the majority of our cases postoperatively, the analysis of risk factors for early mortality has revealed that only patients having a creatine kinase level of more than 1,600 U/L and an MB fraction of 10% or greater are at high risk of an unfavorable outcome. The factors contributing to perioperative infarction have been found to be the presence of left main disease and the absence of well-developed intercoronary col-

TABLE 1.
Follow-up

Parameter	Preoperative (n = 108)	Postoperative			
		1 Month (n = 70)	3 Months (n = 67)	6 Months (n = 51)	12 Months (n = 44)
Angina class	2.56 ± 0.7	0.7 ± 1.1	0.7 ± 1.0	0.8 ± 1.1	0.8 ± 0.9
Angina	100%	33%	35%	40%	46%
TMT					
Duration (min)	5.5 ± 3	6.5 ± 3.4	6.5 ± 3.4	8 ± 3.7	9.7 ± 4.0 ($P < 0.008$)
Workload (METs)	3.6 ± 1.7	3.7 ± 2.1	4.3 ± 2.3	5.4 ± 2.6	6.0 ± 3.4 ($P < 0.005$)
MUGA LVEF(%)	44.7 ± 10.5	42.2 ± 11.7	45.6 ± 18	46 ± 11.6	42 ± 11.7

Abbreviations: TMT, treadmill test; *METs,* metabolic equivalents; *MUGA,* multiple gated acquisition (blood pool image); *LVEF,* left ventricular ejection fraction.

laterals. Additionally, patients with impaired left ventricular function (mean pulmonary artery pressure, > 21 mm Hg) were found to be at a higher risk of early death. Such patients with an "unprotectned myocardium" (left main disease and poorly developed collaterals) and compromised left ventricular function can be salvaged using a combined approach of TMLR with CABG to at least one important vessel. Such patients often need endarterectomies, and even though the long-term patency rate of these grafts are suboptimal, they act as a support to the lased territory and improve the early postoperative outcome.

TMLR COMBINED WITH CORONARY BYPASS AND ENDARTERECTOMY

In group 3, 44 patients needed an endarterectomy of at least one vessel, and significantly, 18 patients needed multiple-vessel endarterectomies and 24 patients needed an endarterectomy of the LAD artery. These patients with severe diffuse coronary artery disease with ungraftable vessels have been denied an opportunity for revascularization. Apart from disabling persistent refractory angina, there is a risk of recurrent multiple infarctions and loss of valuable viable myocardium. Consequently, left ventricular dysfunction develops, and these patients end up on a transplant waiting list. By extending the indications for CABG with endarterectomy and combining these procedures with TMLR, we have been able to achieve adequate revascularization and encouraging results in these patients. The early mortality is comparable to that occurring in patients who undergo isolated CABG and endarterectomy or isolated TMLR. Analysis of early follow-up studies showed a significant reduction in angina in 80% of patients; long-term follow-up is awaited.

MECHANISMS RESPONSIBLE FOR CLINICAL BENEFIT

The exact mechanism by which TMLR improves perfusion and relieves symptoms is unknown, and several theories have been proposed. The placebo effect theory is discredited by the fact that those who had isolated TMLR continue to be symptom free even after 2 to 3 years, whereas a placebo effect is unlikely to persist beyond 6 months. The alternative theory based on reptilian circulatory dynamics states that these endocardially based channels may provide a direct pathway for blood into the intramyocardial sinusoidal plexus, an integral component of intramyocardial microcirculation. This concept is derived from reptilian circulatory dynamics in which 90% of myocardial blood flow is derived from endocardial channels. Berwing et al.,[15] studying these channels by means of coronary angiography and myocardial contrast echocardiography, have demonstrated functional evidence of long-term patency in the human beating heart. However, histopathologic studies have failed to conclusively demonstrate the patency and endothelialization of channels and their communication with sinusoids.[16,17]

Another theory is based on neoangiogenesis induced by thermal and mechanical stimuli. Laser-induced thermal stimuli may lead to vascular angiogenic "growth factor–like" molecules that may potentiate the microcirculation. TMLR has been shown to stimulate angiogenesis in the porcine and canine myocardium. Studying the response in animal experiments, Malekan et al.[18] have concluded that it represents a nonspecific response to tissue injury. Based on their experiments using a canine model of chronic ischemia, Yamamato et al.[19] have concluded that TMLR stimulates angiogenesis, and that the new vessels persist at least 2 months and are capable of mediating an improvement in myocardial blood flow.

In our experience, patients have benefited symptomatically, and the positive trend in terms of relief of angina has continued at 1- and 2-year follow-up. Moreover, they have shown statistically significant improvement in the duration of exercise as well as the metabolic equivalents achieved on treadmill testing performed 6 to 12 months after the procedure. This observation may support the theory of laser-induced neovascularization that develops with time and provides benefits to the myocardium.

FUTURE DIRECTIONS

Cardiologists have begun performing catheter-based TMLR, in which the myocardium is assessed from the left ventricular cavity. The channels are created from the endocardial surface using Ho:YAG and Xe:Cl lasers. Percutaneous TMLR might help to differentiate whether the symptomatic relief provided by surgical TMLR is indeed a placebo effect associated with thoracotomy.

Recently, patients with coronary allograft vasculopathy have been treated with TMLR. Until now, these patients with diffuse coronary artery disease have had retransplantation as their only option, and TMLR may become an effective alternate mode of therapy.[20] In fact, prophylactic TMLR on marginal donor hearts has been proposed to manage accelerated coronary atherosclerosis. Gene transfer techniques to enhance angiogenesis may be used synergistically with TMLR. Sayeed Shah et al.[21] have suggested that nonviral gene transfer at sites of TMLR is feasible, and thermal injury associated with TMLR may enhance both the efficacy and degree of myocardial transgene expression.

SUMMARY

TMLR is effective as an isolated procedure in patients with ungraftable vessels and is a useful adjunct to CABG in patients with diffuse and small-vessel disease requiring endarterectomies. The optimal subset of patients who will benefit from isolated TMLR are those primarily with angina rather than congestive failure, who have protected myocardium and uncompromised left ventricular function.

REFERENCES

1. Mirhoseini M, Shelgikar S, Cayton MM: New concepts in the revascularization of the myocardium. *Ann Thorac Surg* 45:415-420, 1988.
2. Beck CS: The development of a new blood supply to the heart by operation. *Ann Surg* 102:801-813, 1935.
3. Vineberg AM: Clinical and experimental studies in the treatment of coronary artery insufficiency by internal mammary artery implant. *J Int Coll Surg* 22:502-518, 1954.
4. Massimo C, Baffi L: Myocardial revascularization by a new method of carrying blood directly from the left ventricular cavity into the coronary circulation. *J Thorac* 3:257-264, 1957.
5. Sen PK, Udwadia TE, Kinare SG, et al: Transmyocardial acupuncture: A new concept to myocardial revascularisation. *J Thorac Cardiovasc Surg* 50:181-189, 1965.
6. Walter P, Hundeshagen H, Borst HG: Treatment of acute myocardial infarction by transmural blood supply from the ventricular cavity. *Eur Surg Res* 3:130-138, 1971.
7. Jansen ED, Frenz M, Kadipasaoglu KA, et al: Laser-tissue interaction during transmyocardial laser revascularization. *Ann Thorac Surg* 63:640-647, 1997.
8. Horvath KA, Mannting F, Cummings N, et al: Transmyocardial laser revascularisation: Operative techniques and clinical results at two years. *J Thorac Cardiovasc Surg* 111:1047-1053, 1996.
9. Horvath KA, Cohn LH, Cooley DA, et al: Transmyocardial laser revascularisation: Results of a multicenter trial with transmyocardial laser revascularisation used as sole therapy for end stage coronary artery disease. *J Thorac Cardiovasc Surg* 113:645-654, 1997.
10. Satyaprasad V, Madhu Sankar N, Arumugam SB, et al: Transmyocardial laser revascularisation: A new concept in the treatment of coronary artery disease. *Indian Heart J* 47:49-51, 1995.
11. Allen KB, Fudge TL, Sellinger SL, et al: Prospective randomized trial of transmyocardial revascularization versus maximal medical medical management in patients with class IV angina (abstract). *Circulation* 96:564S, 1997.
12. Frazier OH, Cooley DA, Kadipasaoglu KA, et al: Myocardial revascularization with laser: Preliminary findings. *Circulation* 92:58S-65S, 1995.
13. Cooley DA, Frazier OH, Kadipasaoglu KA, et al: Transmyocardial laser revascularization: Clinical experience with twelve-month follow-up. *J Thorac Cardiovasc Surg* 111:791-799, 1996.
14. Lutter G, Saurbier B, Nitsche E, et al: Transmyocardial laser revascularisation in patients with unstable angina and low ejection fraction. *Eur J Cardiothorac Surg* 13:21-26, 1998.

15. Berwing K, Hoyersweda K, Bauer EP, et al: Functional evidence of long-term channel patency after transmyocardial laser revascularisation (abstract). *Circulation* 96:564S, 1997.

16. Krabatsch T, Schaper F, Leder L, et al: Histological findings after transmyocardial laser revascularisation. *J Card Surg* 11:326-331, 1996.

17. Burkhoff D, Fisher PE, Apfelbaum M, et al: Histologic appearance of transmyocardial channels after 4½ weeks. *Ann Thorac Surg* 61:1532-1535, 1996.

18. Malekan IL, Reynolds CA, Kelly ST, et al: Angiogenesis in transmyocardial laser revascularisation: A nonspecific response to injury (abstract). *Circulation* 96:564S, 1996.

19. Yamamato N, Kohmoto T, Gu A, et al: Transmyocardial revascularisation enhances angiogenesis in a canine model of chronic ischaemia (abstract). *Circulation* 96:563S, 1997.

20. March RJ, Guynn T: Cardiac allograft vasculopathy: The potential role for transmyocardial laser revascularization. *J Heart Lung Transplant* 14:242S-246S, 1995.

21. Sayeed Shah U, Mann MJ, Reul RM, et al: Gene transfer in porcine myocardium with transmyocardial laser revascularisation (abstract). *Circulation* 96:482S, 1997.

CHAPTER 4

Cardiac Cell Transplantation: The Autologous Skeletal Myoblast Implantation for Myocardial Regeneration

Ray Chu-Jeng Chiu, M.D., Ph.D.
Professor and Chairman, Division of Cardiothoracic Surgery, McGill University; Director, Division of Cardiothoracic Surgery, McGill University Health Centre, Montreal, Quebec, Canada

With the dawn of the 21st century approaching, one wonders what cardiac surgery will be like in the next millennium. With the advances and convergence of imaging, computing, and robotic technologies, the *cyber-surgery* of the next decade will likely make current minimally invasive cardiac surgery look rather primitive.[1] We can also expect the steady progress of recent years in areas such as gene therapy, including the development of transgenic animals for xenograft and various mechanical cardiac prostheses, will be projected into the future, thereby enriching the armamentarium of cardiac surgeons. These new technologies will have to demonstrate their efficacy in prolonging the high-quality adjusted life expectancy of our patients. In addition, the cost efficiency of these advances will have to be demonstrated, in view of the demography of our aging population and the finite societal resources available for health care.[2]

TISSUE ENGINEERING

With this in mind, the recent rapid development in the science and technology of tissue engineering is of considerable interest.

The term *tissue engineering* is generally applied to the technology in which a body part is constructed and manufactured in vitro using, as the constituents, cellular and extracellular substrates similar to those found in vivo. Such manufactured tissue is then implanted to replace or to supplement the damaged counterpart in the body of a patient. A common approach is to grow a number of cell populations over a biodegradable polymer scaffold under cell culture conditions. Upon implantation the scaffold is absorbed, and the implant is integrated into the host tissue. Because the substitute tissue is produced outside of the body, this approach can be considered *in vitro tissue engineering*. Currently, a product of in vitro tissue engineering—namely, artificial skin—is already approved by the U.S. Food and Drug Administration for clinical use, and laboratory studies are ongoing to tissue engineer cardiac valves,[3] vascular conduits, etc.

In contrast, *in vivo tissue engineering* is a process by which the body constitutes and develops new tissue after implantation of cells or other substrates. An example of this in clinical use is the hematologic stem cell administration to reconstitute bone marrow after aggressive chemotherapy for cancer. Such cells may, under proper conditions, differentiate into mature cells that are of therapeutic value to the patient. The *cardiac cell transplantation* discussed in this chapter is therefore an in vivo tissue engineering of the myocardium carried out to repair the damaged heart muscle, i.e., cellular cardiomyoplasty.[4]

CELLULAR CARDIOMYOPLASTY

Unlike salamanders, which can regenerate and repair damaged myocardium, the cardiac muscles of postnatal mammals (including humans) are terminally differentiated and have minimal or no capacity to proliferate and repair damaged cardiac muscle fibers. When cardiac muscles are lost through apoptosis or necrosis (as with heart failure and after coronary artery occlusions), the muscle fibers are permanently lost or are replaced by scar tissue. The remaining muscle fibers can compensate only by hypertrophy or elongation. Thus, the idea of replenishing lost cardiac myocytes is of interest. This has been attempted by manipulating genes to awaken the proliferative capacity of the native cardiac muscle and by implanting cells and allowing them to differentiate and grow into new cardiac muscle fibers. In spite of considerable advances in our knowledge of genetic mechanisms of the cardiac muscle cells, genetic engineering has not successfully been used to regenerate cardiac muscle thus far. In contrast, cell transplantation has been successful in growing new cardiac muscle in vivo in a number of animal models.

FETAL CARDIAC MYOCYTE IMPLANTATION

There are a number of cell populations that can potentially be considered candidates for implantation to achieve myocardial regeneration. The most obvious one is that of fetal cardiac myocytes. These cells are capable of mitotic division and proliferation in utero, and they develop into mature cardiac muscle fibers. Fetal cardiac myocytes have been isolated, cultured in vitro, labeled with cell markers, and implanted into normal or injured adult myocardial tissue. Several investigators have demonstrated that these cells can grow and differentiate into adult cardiac myocytes and that they are capable of forming desmosome cell junctions with native cardiac myocytes, which are histologically recognizable as intercalated discs.[5] In certain animal models with cryoinjured myocardium, such neomyocardium grown from implanted fetal cardiac myocytes have been shown to improve cardiac function. Clinically, however, there are two obvious disadvantages of using fetal cardiac myocytes for this purpose. First, there are ethical and logistic difficulties in obtaining a sufficient amount of fetal hearts, which are the source for such donor cells, when they are to be used therapeutically for patients with heart failure. Furthermore, fetal cardiac myocyte implantation is in fact the transference of allografts, which means that the recipient requires immunosuppression similar to that required by patients who receive organ transplantation from another individual. Thus, although fetal cardiac myocyte implantation is of considerable biological interest, its clinical applicability would likely be limited. It should be noted also that there is evidence that transplantation of mature cardiac myocytes will not be successful.

MYOBLAST CELL-LINE IMPLANTATION

Another type of cells favored by cell biologists as donor cells for myocardial implantation are the established cell-line myoblasts, such as C2 C12 cells.[6] The use of such cells is convenient to investigators because the cells can be purchased and perpetuated in culture in the laboratory. C2 C12 cells were originally derived from skeletal myoblasts, but their phenotype had been somewhat altered to allow them to divide and grow indefinitely. Thus, although the cell-lines are convenient for laboratory use, they acquire oncogenic potential when implanted into recipients because they have been immortalized in culture. Again, experiments using myoblasts of established cell-line myoblasts are of scientific interest but may not be suitable for therapeutic use.

SATELLITE CELL IMPLANTATION

To avoid these pitfalls for clinical application, several investigators have undertaken a different approach by using, as donor cells, the autologous skeletal myoblasts of adult animals, which are known as *satellite cells.* It is hypothesized that such cells, under proper conditions, can undergo *milieu-dependent differentiation* to express cardiac myocyte phenotypes after the cells are implanted into the myocardium.[7] Because these are autologous cells, no immunosuppression will be necessary, and the difficulties of using fetal tissue can be avoided. Unlike the established cell-line myoblasts, these primary myoblasts will not divide indefinitely to pose the risk of malignancy. Because of such apparent advantages for therapeutic use, the following sections of this chapter will focus on this particular approach, discussing its biological background, experimental findings to date, and possible future clinical applications. Readers who are interested in a broader review of cardiac cell transplantation are recommended to consult more extensive reviews recently published.[8,9]

BIOLOGICAL BASIS OF SATELLITE CELL (SKELETAL MYOBLAST) TRANSPLANTATION FOR MYOCARDIAL REGENERATION
PROLIFERATION AND DIFFERENTIATION OF MYOCYTES
Responses of Cardiac Versus Skeletal Muscles to Injury

The cellular acquisition of specialized functions and the irreversible arrest from a cell cycle are termed *terminal differentiation.*[10] The molecular mechanisms responsible for terminal differentiation are not fully understood. Cardiomyocytes maintain their ability to proliferate only as they proceed through their initial stages of differentiation during embryonic development. Shortly after birth, differentiated myocytes permanently withdraw from the cell cycle and the cardiac myocytes lose their ability to proliferate; growth of the heart occurs mainly by the hypertrophy of pre-existing cardiomyocytes.[11,12]

Skeletal muscle, on the other hand, can regenerate and effectively restore its function after an injury. New skeletal muscle fiber formation from the ends of existing fibers and the reuniting of transected fibers are well documented.[13] The discovery of skeletal muscle satellite cells in the early 1960s led to the identification of the events leading to skeletal muscle regeneration.[14] These satellite cells, normally dormant in adults, behave as embryonic myoblasts that avidly participate in skeletal muscle regeneration. They are distinct from the multinucleated skeletal muscle fiber and retain the capacity for mitotic cycling in the event of injury, which is the main stimulus for its activation.[15] In contrast, regenerative capacity has not been demonstrated in adult cardiac muscle after injury. Recent studies show that a rapid switch of cardiac myocytes from hyperplasia to hypertrophy occurred during early postnatal development. Cardiomyocyte DNA synthesis in normal and injured adult mammalian heart tissue is extremely rare when myocyte nuclei can be reliably identified. In a rat model of myocardial injury, it was shown that the potential for DNA synthesis in cardiac muscle cells progressively declines soon after birth.[16] After cell death occurs, myocardial repair consists of connective tissue proliferation and scar formation, which inevitably leads to loss of function and progressive heart failure. This inability to repair after an incidence of injury has been attributed to the absence of stem cells in mammalian cardiac muscle. The use of autologous myogenic stem cells can potentially restore the cardiac function of an injured heart by replenishing its critical muscle mass. The approach described below attempts to use skeletal muscle myoblasts as the source of progenitor cells to regenerate damaged myocardial tissue.

Biology of Satellite Cells (Skeletal Myoblasts)

Satellite cells have the ability to divide and give rise to differentiated cells and new satellite cells. They also have the ability to cycle in vitro.[17] Thus, these cells can be seen as stem cells. Under electron microscopy, satellite cells appear indistinguishable by their position beneath the basal lamina of the skeletal muscle fibers, but unlike the muscle fiber nuclei, they lie outside sarcolemma. Adult satellite cells revert to their active form after being stimulated by disease, ischemia, exercise, or direct trauma.[18] Satellite cell nuclei make up about 5% of all the nuclei in the muscle fiber. This has been confirmed in animals as well as in humans.[19] Within the basal lamina, satellite cells have the ability to migrate toward the injury site.[20] This suggests the possible role of muscle injury in releasing factors that can activate satellite cells and guide them to the injury site. A question that has been raised is whether satellite cells are identical to embryonic myoblasts. Much of the evidence available suggests that, although satellite cells resemble embryonic myoblasts, the former is most likely a subpopulation of the latter. Analysis of muscle regeneration has shown that muscle satellite cells synthesize embryonic isoforms of myosin and tropomyosin.[21] This suggests that in regenerated muscle originating from satellite cells the differentiation sequence is similar to that of embryonic muscle. Interestingly, using tritiated thymidine labeling and radioautography, it was found that myoblasts and satellite cells were able to recognize each other and fuse to form hybrid myotubules when cocultured.[22]

Localized injury to the myofiber activates satellite cells positioned not only in close vicinity to the damaged area. Studies on myogenic transcription factors have shown that, in cases of injury to skeletal muscle, the appearance of these early myogenic markers precedes the mitotic activity of satellite cells. Furthermore, these factors became expressed even in the satellite cells farther away from the injured site. Satellite cells possess migratory ability that can be a valuable feature in recruiting neighboring myogenic cells to repair injured skeletal muscle fibers.[23]

Satellite cells extend their repairing ability to postnatal myofibers. Studies on patients with Duchenne's muscular dystrophy showed that skeletal myoblasts of heterogenic origin can fuse with the host myofibers and contribute to the expression of structural protein. When myoblasts of genetically different animal species were cocultured in vitro, muscle cells of both species contributed to the formation of *mosaic* myofibers.[24] In addition, it has been shown that satellite cells are able to withstand an ischemic environment for up to 18 to 24 hours, a feature that is valuable for cells involved in muscle repair.[25]

Cellular Differentiation Pathways

Cell differentiation and phenotypic expression may follow three basic pathways. Most cells used in cellular transplantation, such as fetal cardiac myocytes, follow the *lineage-dependent* differentiation pathway. This implies that cell commitment to a certain phenotype is determined during the early stages of embryonic development. Such cells will faithfully develop into lineage-predetermined tissue regardless of their environment. In contrast, *transdifferentiation* implies that even terminally differentiated cells have the ability to alter their phenotypes.[26] This phenomenon has been well documented in skeletal muscle transformation used in the dynamic cardiomyoplasty procedure,[27] in which fatigue-prone type II fast-twitch muscle fibers are converted into fatigue-resistant type I slow-twitch fibers by low frequency electrical stimulation. Moreover, this process does not require cytokinesis or cell division, the latter of which was previously thought to be uniformly compulsory for the cell to change its phenotype. The third pathway postulates that the major determinant in cell differentiation can be in the cellular environment. This cell differentiation pathway is known as *milieu-dependent* differentiation.[28] For example, it has been demonstrated that myoblasts, if exposed to a bone morphological factor that is a member of a transforming growth factor (TGF) family, undergo phenotypic transformation into osteoblasts.[29] These and other examples lend support to the plausible idea that satellite cells, if introduced into the cardiac environment, might be influenced in their differentiation pathway to express the phenotype of the cardiac myocytes. It has been suggested that the first and most important factor necessary for embryonic cells to be committed to the myogenic lineage is the so-called *community effect*.[30] Somite embryonic cells, which are not myogenic precursor cells, can be influenced to commit to enter a myogenic lineage if they are cultured with other cells from the trunk in 3-dimensional conditions. It appears that a critical number of mesodermal cells are required to commence the differentiation process. This suggests that cell-to-cell interaction, as well as specific spatial structures, play a significant modulatory role in muscle differentiation. Indeed, there are numerous reports indicating that cell culture density affects cell commitment to a certain phenotype. Studies with in vitro embryonic chick mesenchymal cells showed that culture density is the primary factor that determines the phenotype of cultured cells. When mesenchymal cells are plated at a high density and consequently have ample cell-to-cell contact, they consistently produce chondrocyte-like cells that synthesize type II collagen and keratin sulfate proteoglycan. When cell-to-cell contact is reduced by decreasing cell culture density, the culture shifts to osteoblast formation with the expression of bone alkaline phosphatase and cell response to parathyroid hormone.[31]

Implicit to this approach is the idea that as the injured cardiac muscle degenerates, it may provide the environment that can specifically induce the differentiation of satellite cells implanted into the myocardium. It has been shown that transplanted fetal cardiac myoblasts within the myocardium may form electrical links to host cells through gap junctions in addition to making physical connections through desmosomes.[32] If similar connections can be demonstrated between the neomyocardium derived from satellite cells and the native cardiac muscle, it is highly likely that the neomyocardium can be functionally integrated and become clinically useful to repair injured myocardium in patients with heart failure. These issues will be discussed further below.

REGULATION OF MUSCLE DIFFERENTIATION

In addition to direct cell-to-cell communication, a number of other mechanisms are known to influence cell differentiation. These include genetic control, various growth factors, and extra-cellular matrix. Elucidation of control mechanisms of myoblast differentiation may enable the development of a strategy to direct the differentiation process such that the desired phenotype may be expressed for therapeutic use.

Genetic Controls

The development of skeletal muscle cells is determined by the expression of genes encoding myogenic transcription factors of the myogenic determination factors (MyoD) family, such a Myf-5, MyoD, myogenin (also known as Myf-4), and MRF-4 (also known as Myf-6 or herculin). All of the above proteins belong to the basic-helix-loop-helix (bHLH) superfamily. The proteins of bHLH super-family have been shown to regulate cell fate specifications during embryologic development. The proteins of the MyoD family can activate the whole cascade of skeletal muscle–specific genes in myogenic cells. Furthermore, it has been shown that the same proteins are able to initiate myogenic programs in nonmyogenic cells and convert them into skeletal muscle cells.[33] For example, fibroblasts obtained from the myocardium have been converted into skeletal myocytes in vitro using this technique.

Both cardiac and skeletal muscles are derived from the mesoderm. However, cardiac muscle is formed earlier in the embryogenesis than is skeletal muscle. In the second week of human embryo development, cells from the primitive streak migrate along notochordal process toward prochordal plate. Just rostral to this structure, migrating cells meet and form the cardiogenic area where, by the end of the third week of development, two endothelial heart tubes fuse to form a primitive beating heart tube. The striated muscle cells also differ in the sequence of proliferation and differentiation events. Skeletal myoblast differentiation and expression of muscle proteins commences after the proliferation phase, and these two events are mutually exclusive in time. Meanwhile, fetal cardiac myocytes have the ability to produce structural muscle proteins and to continue to enter the mitotic cell cycle. Despite temporal and spatial differences in their embryologic development, both types of striated muscle share many structural proteins and have identical contractile units. Although there are no known MyoD family members present in the heart muscle, some reports suggest that the α-cardiac actin gene, which is in skeletal muscle regulated by MyoD in conjunction with other factors, appears to be regulated by bHLH proteins in the cardiac muscle as well.[34] Furthermore, muscle enhancer factor-2—a member of the MADS box family of transcription factors that participates in the initiation of the myogenic program in skeletal myoblasts—has been found to participate in the transcription of at least two cardiac muscle genes (cardiac troponin T and myosin light chain-2).[35]

Even with an advancing knowledge in the embryogenesis of striated muscles, it is still difficult to predict whether it is indeed possible to coax skeletal myoblasts to transdifferentiate into cardiac myocytes. Thus, at present, satellite cell transplantation for myocardial regeneration is largely confined to observational descriptive studies, and mechanistic investigation is still to be pursued in the future.

Growth Factors

The growth, development, and differentiation processes of both cardiac and skeletal muscle cells are influenced and directed by the effect of the growth factors present in their environment. Studies performed in the mid-1980s showed that a crushed adult muscle is a potent mitogen for satellite cells. It has been demonstrated that crushed muscle extract contains such mitogenic factors as transferrin, basic fibroblast growth factor (bFGF), insulin-like growth factor (IGF-1), platelet-derived growth factor (PDGF-BB), and an uncharacterized heparin-binding factor that is able to stimulate muscle cell proliferation as well.[36]

Fibroblast growth factors, both acidic (αFGF) and basic, are shown to stimulate myogenic cell division and to repress or delay the terminal differentiation. Of particular interest are data that a growth factor strongly mitogenic for chicken skeletal myoblasts has been isolated from rat, chicken, sheep, and cow atrial and ventricular heart tissue extracts. This mitogen has been identified as bFGF. It was noted that bFGF was localized in close relationship with specific structures of cardiac myocytes, such as nuclei, basal membrane, and intercalated discs.[37]

αFGF is also expressed in abundance in cardiac myocytes during embryogenesis. It has been shown that αFGF is produced by heart muscle cells and deposited within the surrounding extracellular matrix where it can act in paracrine fashion. Data demonstrating that αFGF expression is highest in fetal and early neonatal ventricles support the role of αFGF in capillary angiogenesis as well as in ventricular maturation and remodeling in the cardiac development.[38]

TGF-β is known as a potent inhibitor of myoblast differentiation. When added to the myogenic cell culture, it inhibits myoblast fusion into myotubules and other biochemical parameters of differentiation.[39]

There are 3 isoforms of mammalian TGF-β, and all of them are expressed in the heart. Cardiac myocytes express three TGF-β receptors, and all three TGF-βs play important roles in the organogenesis, the induction of the mesodermal layer, and the expression of cardiac muscle cell phenotype.[40] It has also been shown that TGF-β plays an important role in the cascade of events initiated by the functional overload.[41] Of interest are data revealing that contrary to skeletal myoblasts, in which TGF-β inhibits myogenic gene activation and halts cells in the G1 phase of the cell cycle, TGF-β activates the whole group of fetal cardiac genes, such as skeletal α-actin, β-myosin heavy chain, atrial natriuretic factor, and smooth muscle α-actin in cardiac myocytes.[41]

IGFs type I (IGF-I) and type II (IGF-II) play an important role in the activation of the myogenic program and the proliferation and differentiation of muscle cells. Myoblasts transduced with IGF-I gene driven by skeletal α-actin promoter in C2 C12 muscle cell line demonstrated an enhanced expression of myogenic transcription factors, as well as contractile proteins.[42]

IGF-II accumulates during myoblast differentiation. This growth factor has the ability to down-regulate IGF-I receptor and may blunt the myogenic effect of IGF-I, thus switching muscle cells toward the differentiation pathway.[43]

Thus, although our understanding of the effects of various growth factors is not complete, they clearly do affect the microenvironment of the myoblasts and guide their differentiation.

Extracellular Matrix

Another important component of cellular milieu is the extracellular matrix (ECM), which provides a substrate for cell attachment as well as signal transduction through the specific receptors to the cell. Spatial and temporal expression of the different components of ECM are thought to influence organogenesis dramatically. Multi-potent mesenchymal cells derived from chick tail buds have been shown to differentiate into a variety of tissues if exposed to different ECM components in vitro.[44] In muscle differentiation, it is known that a number of components of muscle basal laminae can affect myoblast differentiation and regeneration. These components include laminin, proteoglycans, entactin (or nidogen), tenascin, and collagen type IV. Specifically, collagen type VIII has been found to be expressed during cardiogenesis in mice, and it is implicated to be involved in the differentiation of cardiac myocytes and the formation of cardiac valves.[45]

The ECM sites rich in fibronectin serve as guides for migrating embryonic cells during organogenesis. In adult mammals, production of fibronectin increases after injury to tissues. Therefore, it appears that fibronectin plays an important role in the tissue regeneration process.[46]

Integrins are found not only on the cell surface in contact with the ECM proteins but also at the cell-to-cell interface. Integrin $\alpha_5\beta_1$ is also developmentally regulated during myogenesis, because enhanced binding of this integrin and its ligand are shown to interfere with the cell migration and morphogenesis of myotubules. After the differentiation of the muscle cells, the localization pattern of this integrin is changed, permitting muscle cells to acquire structural changes as myogenesis proceeds.[47]

Other cell adhesion molecules, such as neural cell adhesion molecules (NCAMs), are found at the cell-to-cell interface as well. NCAMs are detected in somites early, even before the formation of myotome compartments. Cells in the myotomes as well as adult myoblasts express two major isoforms on myoblasts, namely the 180-kD and the 140-kD transmembrane NCAM isoforms.

Overexpression experiments have shown that both isoforms promote myoblast fusion.[48]

Cell-to-cell interaction during embryogenesis is regulated by cadherins, calcium-dependent cell adhesion molecules. M-cadherin production is downregulated after birth. However, this protein reappears on regenerating myoblasts and fades away after myotubule formation.[49]

In summary, the attempts to regenerate myocardial tissue by satellite cell implantation are based on the hypothesis that the complex environment within myocardial tissue, elucidated in part above, may allow the milieu-dependent differentiation to take place, coaxing implanted skeletal myoblasts to transdifferentiate into muscle fibers that express many or all of the phenotypic characteristics of cardiac myocytes.

EXPERIMENTAL MODELS AND METHODS
ANIMAL SPECIES AND MODELS

A number of animal species and experimental models have been used to study primary skeletal myoblast implantation into the myocardium. In canine studies, the satellite cells isolated from the anterior tibialis muscle have been injected into the left ventricular wall of the same animal as auto-implants.[50] The removal of the anterior tibialis muscle appeared to cause no obvious dysfunction of the extremities. When using rabbits as the experimental models, investigators have also used autologous primary skeletal myoblasts as the donor cells.[51] When a rat is used as the recipient, another isogenic rat (genetically identical to the recipient) is used as the source of donor cells because of the small size of the animal and because of the ready availability of isogenic animals in this species.[52] As can be seen, all these experiments bypass the question of allograft rejection and the need for immunosuppression after transplantation. Positive results have been obtained in all these animal models, as will be described later.

Because this is a relatively new field of research, many important factors that may affect outcome have not been scrutinized. For example, the number of satellite cells in the skeletal muscle may decrease with age, but to date this issue has not been studied systematically. Whether all the skeletal muscle in the body contains satellite cells similar in quantity and quality needs to be determined. From a clinical point of view, muscles that are important to the normal functioning of the body will clearly not be suitable as the donor tissue. Studies in dynamic cardiomyoplasty have shown that the use of the latissimus dorsi muscle and a number of other thoracic skeletal muscles caused no obvious functional impairment to patients.[27] This is not surprising, considering these same muscles have been used for reconstructive surgery, for coverage of the infected sternal wound, and for filling of infected intrathoracic space. Thus, these muscles would be potential donor tissues for harvesting the autologous satellite cells.

SATELLITE CELL ISOLATION AND CULTURE

Immediately after the donor muscle explantation, excessive connective tissue and fascia are removed from the specimen by mechanical dissection. Using a series of enzymatic digestion and centrifugation procedures, the satellite cells are isolated. Detailed technical procedures have been described by various investigators and readers interested in these details are referred to the references cited.[50-52] Generally, the cell pellets obtained after such an isolation procedure contain, in addition to satellite cells, some fibroblasts. Whether the presence of fibroblasts in the implant cell population is useful or harmful is not known at present. The donor cell population can be purified to reduce the proportion of fibroblasts using density centrifugation or gel column to remove the majority of the fibroblasts and cells other than the satellite cells. The viability of isolated satellite cells can be assessed by trypan blue exclusion test. The isolated cells are cultured in vitro using an appropriate growth medium. By splitting the culture for passaging repeatedly, the plating density of cells can be controlled. As will be discussed later, the culture cell density in vitro may be one of the determinants of phenotype expression after the implantation of these cells into the myocardium.

At present, the proportion of satellite cells in the culture may be estimated through observation of spindle-shaped satellite cells in comparison with other cells that may appear polygonal (Fig 1). There have been no reports of the use of phenotype molecular markers to identify satellite cells in culture. One reliable method to confirm the presence of satellite cells in culture is to allow cells in one of the culture plates to continue multiplying without splitting. When high density is reached, the satellite cells would become confluent and form multinucleated striated muscle fibers (Fig 2). Although not quantitatively useful, this assures that functioning satellite cells are present. The amount of splitting of the cultures and the length of the culture period will depend on the desired culture cell density and the total quantity of cells to be made available for implantation. Experimentally, to be able to trace the fate of the implanted cells, the satellite cells are labeled while in culture so that they can be identified even after their in vivo proliferation and differentiation. In the therapeutic use of cell transplantation, such cell labeling would not be required.

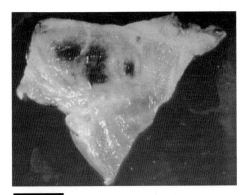

FIGURE 3.

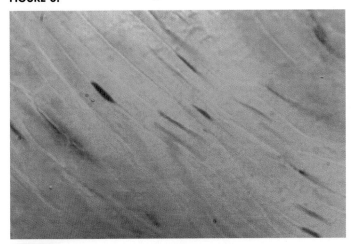

FIGURE 4.

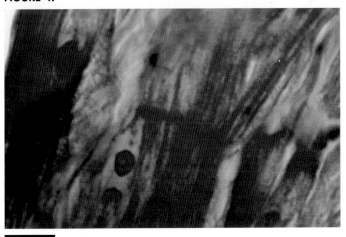

FIGURE 5.

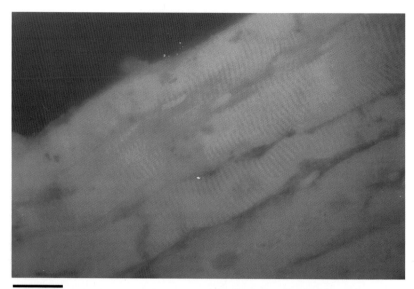

FIGURE 6.

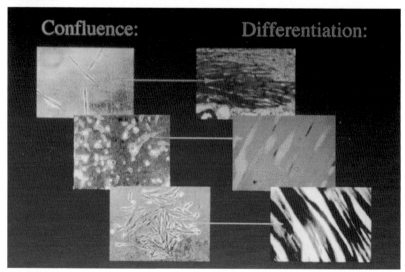

FIGURE 7.

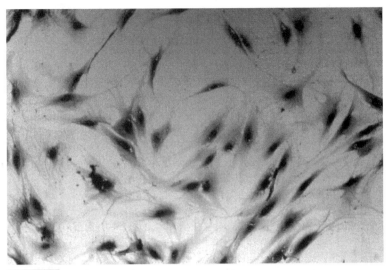

FIGURE 1.
Satellite cells in culture.

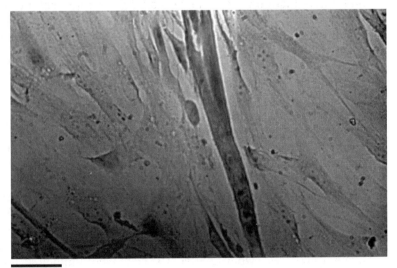

FIGURE 2.
Satellite cells in culture that fused and differentiated into a multinucleated striated muscle fiber.

CELL-LABELING TECHNIQUES

Several cell-labeling techniques have been used by various investigators. One of the common labeling techniques is the use of tritiated thymidine, which would be incorporated into cellular DNA during cell division; its radioactivity could be identified later by subjecting the histologic section to radioautographic studies. The results obtained with this technique have been largely unsatisfactory, and it has been speculated that this may be caused by a couple of factors. If the cell continues to divide repeatedly after the incorporation of tritiated thymidine into the DNA, it will be successively diluted such that ultimately the cell will contain radioactivity levels so low that it would be difficult to identify the existence of radioactivity conclusively with radioautography. If one increases the amount of tritiated thymidine sufficiently to reduce dilutional consequence, the radioactivity within the cellular nucleus may be so strong as to be lethal to the cells. Thus, few reports have used tritiated thymidine as the cell marker in satellite cell implantation studies.

The use of reporter gene for cell labeling has been more successful.[50,51] The *Escherichia coli*–derived *lac Z* gene can be transected into satellite cells using liposomes or viral vectors. The *lac Z* gene encodes the production of β-galactosidase, and the enzymatic activity of β-galactosidase in the specimen can be demonstrated by X-Gal stain, which exhibits blue coloring in the labeled cells. Using this technique, a number of investigators have demonstrated the survival and differentiation of satellite cells after their implantation into the myocardium. One of the limitations of using this reporter gene is the relatively low transfection rate, which seems to be better when adenovirus is used as vector rather than the liposomes.[53] Another limitation is the loss of gene expression over time, which may be related to the loss of appropriate promoters.

Another more novel technique for cell labeling is the use of a compound known as DAPI (4',6-diamidino-2-phenylindole), which can bind to DNA and to the protein tubulin to form a fluorescent complex. After the incubation of the satellite cells with DAPI in vitro, virtually all the cells are labeled, which can be confirmed by observing the specimen under a fluorescent microscope. Recently, using such DAPI-labeled cells, investigators have clearly demonstrated that satellite cells implanted into the myocardium can in fact differentiate into fully developed striated muscle fibers, with centrally located nuclei and intercalated discs, both characteristics of cardiac muscle fibers. In contrast, when the labeled cells were implanted into the skeletal muscle, they developed into muscle fibers with multiple labeled nuclei that are peripherally located in the muscle fibers, as seen normally in the skeletal muscles.[52] Thus, the use of effective cell-labeling technique facilitates the confirmation that the observed tissue in fact originated from the implanted cells.

THE MYOCARDIAL INJURY MODELS AND THE ROUTES OF MYOCARDIAL CELL IMPLANTATION

The harvested labeled satellite cells in culture are then ready for implantation into the myocardium. A number of investigators have used a cryoinjury model of the heart, in which a discrete area of the left ventricular muscle was destroyed by applying a cryoprobe at the epicardial surface.[7] Sufficiently long application of the cryoprobe can produce transmural necrosis of the myocardium, later resulting in a homogeneous scar. Implantation of cells within this scar area enables the investigators to identify the new muscle grown from the implanted cells and to separate them from the native myocardium, even without the use of cell labeling, because the new muscle fibers will be surrounded by the scar tissue. However, cryoinjury is an iatrogenic injury model with no clinical counterparts.

A more clinically relevant myocardial injury model can be created by coronary artery ligation.[9] Such a lesion, particularly in dogs with ample native collateral circulation, will be heterologous, with scar tissue intermingled with surviving native muscle fibers. Implantation into such a region would therefore require cell labeling to identify new muscle among the native muscle fibers. It should be noted that creating a myocardial injury model in the recipient animal has two purposes. First, it is an attempt to simulate the clinical condition of using cell implant to treat damaged myocardium. Second, as discussed earlier, muscle damage appears to be the stimulus needed for satellite cell proliferation, migration, and differentiation. It is thought that the myocardial lesion created may also serve this purpose.

Nevertheless, earlier studies using fetal cardiac myocytes have shown that cells implanted by local injection into the myocardium may still differentiate into mature cardiac muscle fibers,[5] and perhaps the trauma of puncture itself may be sufficient to induce satellite cell proliferation and differentiation. With reliable cell-labeling techniques at hand, studies have been successfully carried out with normal hearts in which the cells were implanted by direct injection.[52] The myoblasts can be delivered into the desired site within the ventricular wall by direct needle puncture, either through the epicardial side or from the endocardial side using an endovascular approach. With this technique of implantation, it has been observed that injected cells are centered at the site of injection, with cell density decreasing as the distance from the injection site increases. The pattern is not regular; injected cells may track the interstitial space and planes in their distribution.

Another approach is to deliver the myoblasts through intracoronary injection, resulting in a more homogeneous distribution of myoblasts throughout the layers of the myocardium.[54] In spite of embolizing the coronary artery with these cells, it has been reported that no myocardial infarction ensued, and the myoblasts were reported to be capable of migrating through the vessel wall and surviving and growing outside of the vasculature. This kind of phenomenon has been reported not only in established cell line (C2 C12) myoblasts,[6] but also in primary skeletal myoblasts.[54] In fact, myoblasts have been genetically engineered and injected intravascularly to deliver them to the peripheral tissue for gene therapy, not only because they can sustain good gene expression, but also because of their ability for extravascular migration. Elucidation of this phenomenon and mechanism of myoblast migration through the vascular wall could be an interesting area of research in the future.

THE "WINNING CONDITIONS" IN CELL IMPLANTATION

A number of investigators have experienced perplexing inconsistencies in cardiac cell implantation studies. In some *responders,* the neomyocardium can be clearly demonstrated, whereas in others none could be found. It is likely that this inconsistency is a reflection of the lack of knowledge regarding the optimal implant conditions. For example, cell implantation immediately after the creation of cryoinjuries or ischemic injuries could expose the implanted cells to a ravaging inflammatory response, so that the implanted cells are attacked by phagocytes that pour in to clear up the debris of the necrotic myocardial tissue. Lack of nourishing blood flow sufficient to sustain neomyocardial survival when the cells are implanted into the center of a dense scar may also doom the experiments to failure. Elucidation of these and other factors that may affect the outcome of the implant cells need to be carried out before the procedure can be considered for therapeutic use with reliable reproducibility.

MORPHOLOGICAL FINDINGS
GROSS SPECIMENS

A gross specimen of the heart harvested 4 to 6 weeks after satellite cell implantation into a cryoinjured myocardium reveals brownish tissue at the site of implantation, surrounded by white scar tissue (Fig 3). When the satellite cells implanted were transected with a reporter gene *(lac Z)* in vitro while being cultured, staining of the cardiac specimen with X-Gal revealed the characteristic blue color of β-galactosidase activity at the implant site.[50] The gross specimen of hearts that received satellite cell implantation without creating a cryolesion appeared normal on gross inspection. However, if the satellite cells were labeled with *lac Z* gene, a blue discoloration of the tissue at the implant site indicated the presence of cells derived from the implants.

The distribution of the tissue thought to be derived from implanted satellite cells is determined in part by the technique of

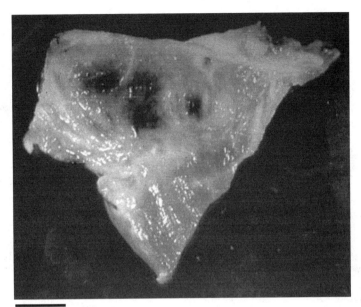

FIGURE 3.
Canine cardiac specimen 4 weeks after implantation of autologous satellite cells into a left ventricular transmural cryoinjury site. The *top* of the picture is epicardium, the *bottom* shows a portion of the normal papillary muscle. The reddish-pink tissue at the center of the whitish scar tissue was the site of satellite cell implantation.

implantation. With injection at one site, the tissue appears to be globus shaped with poorly defined margins. When the cells are implanted into a subepicardial tunnel parallel to the surface of the heart, a layer of brownish tissue sandwiched by white scar can be seen when the implant was made within the zone of the transmural cryoinjury.[50]

HISTOLOGIC STUDIES
The satellite cells that are detached from culture media and implanted into the myocardium initially take the appearance of round cells with large nuclei. They appear to elongate in subsequent days, and they form muscle fibers with striations within 2 to 4 weeks of implantation.[52] Whether there is any species difference in the time course of maturation and differentiation of satellite cells is at present unknown.

Although all tissues derived from implanted satellite cells have been reported to be striated muscle fibers, the histologic features vary, expressing the characteristics of different phenotypes of a striated muscle.[55] In some, the striated muscle tissue showed muscle fibers that do not branch and that contain multiple dense, elon-

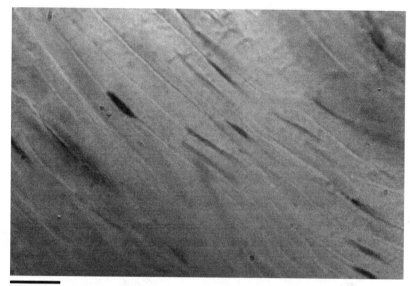

FIGURE 4.

Histology (hematoxylin-eosin stain) of tissue grown at the implant site after autologous implantation of canine satellite cells into the myocardium. In this specimen, the striated muscle fibers show spindle-shaped, peripherally located nuclei with no evidence of intercalated disks. These features are representative of skeletal muscle fibers.

gated, and peripherally located nuclei, which are seen normally in skeletal muscle fibers. In such tissues, intercalated disks are absent (Fig 4). In contrast, other specimens showed branching striated muscle fibers, containing intercalated disks and vesicular, centrally located nuclei, which are normally found in cardiac muscle fibers (Fig 5). To make the situation more complex, in one study in which satellite cells were implanted into a cryoinjured myocardium, the muscle fibers growing at the center of the scar tissue showed histologic characteristics of skeletal muscle, whereas those in the periphery of the scar tissue adjacent to surviving native myocardial tissue showed the appearance of immature cardiac myocytes.[51] In another study, the investigators reported the observation of a mosaic skeletal muscle fiber, which consisted of branching striated muscle fibers without intercalated disks and contained both multiple elongated, peripherally located nuclei and vesicular, centrally located nuclei within the same fiber.[55] Thus, current data suggests that, depending on implant conditions, either skeletal muscle, cardiac muscle, or both could develop from implanted satellite cells. The speculation regarding which implant conditions may affect phenotypic outcome of the new muscle fibers will be discussed below.

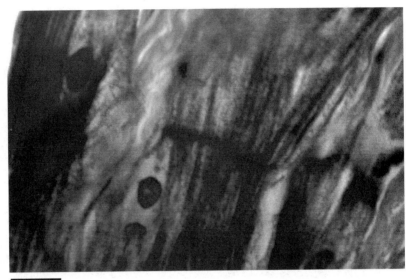

FIGURE 5.
Another specimen obtained from the site of autologous canine satellite cell implantation into a cryoinjured myocardium. This histologic section (Masson trichome stain) shows blue scar tissue containing striated muscle fibers with clear intercalated disks. The oval and vesicular centrally located nuclei resemble those of cardiac myocytes. (Information courtesy of Race L. Kao, Ph.D., East Tennessee University, Johnson City, Tenn.)

IMMUNOHISTOCHEMICAL AND ELECTRON MICROSCOPIC STUDIES

The ultrastructural and immunohistochemical studies designed to identify phenotype molecular markers for regenerated myocytes are so far scarce but are currently under intensive investigation. Specimens obtained from both the implantation of primary skeletal myoblasts, namely satellite cells, and of C2 C12 myoblast–derived cell lines have been examined for Connexin 43 expression. Connexin 43 is a constituent protein of intercalated disks and desmosome junctions and is found to be positive in new muscle fibers histologically resembling cardiac muscle fibers (Fig 6). These new muscle fibers and their cell junctions appear to align in parallel with the native muscle fibers, and one may speculate that this could be in response to the sheer stress of the contracting myocardium. Electron microscopic examination of the cell junction between the implanted C2 C12 cell and adjacent native cardiac myocyte revealed well-developed spot desmosomes at points of contact between these cells. Interestingly, in spite of the establishment of such connection, the implanted cells showed smaller and fewer mitochondria compared with the adjacent cardiac myocytes.[6] Thus, the formation of such junctional apparatus may not necessarily indicate total cardiac myocyte phenotype expression in the implanted cells.

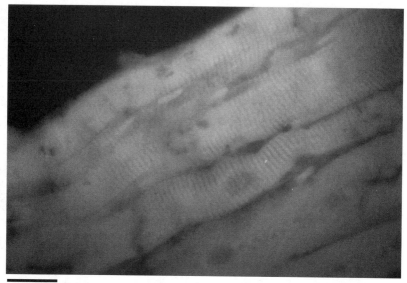

FIGURE 6.

New tissue that formed within canine myocardium after autotransplantation of satellite cells, which was labeled with DAPI during culture and before implantation. Under fluorescent microscopy, labeled cells become fluorescent. Immunohistochemistry of this specimen also demonstrates the presence of Connexin 43, a protein constituent of the intercalated disk. Thus, this microphotography shows labeled striated muscle fibers with clear intercalated disk and centrally located nuclei similar to those seen in cardiac muscle fibers. (Information courtesy of Race L. Kao, Ph.D., East Tennessee University, Johnson City, Tenn.)

In addition to the expression of a cardiac gap junction protein (Connexin 43), the co-expression of the slow-twitch/cardiac protein phospholamban in implanted C2 C12 cells has also been reported. Phospholamban is normally seen only in cardiac myocytes, whereas the skeletal muscle sarcoplasmic reticular marker *SERCA1* is expressed in skeletal muscles. Thus, the co-expression of these two proteins suggests that some aspects of the cardiac milieu may have altered the developmental program of the implanted skeletal myoblast derived cells,[6] resulting in a mosaic myocyte at the molecular level.

HYPOTHESIS ON MODULATORS OF MYOBLAST DIFFERENTIATION

The findings described above, which indicate that adult skeletal myoblasts isolated and cultured in vitro—when implanted into the myocardium—may differentiate into striated muscle fibers of various phenotypes (cardiac, skeletal, and even mosaic), suggests that the differentiation of such cells can be influenced by the experimental conditions. For many years, it has been known that skeletal myoblasts cultured on decalcified bone matrix could differentiate into chondrocytes. Thus, it is apparent that, although satellite cells under normal conditions will undergo lineage-dependent differentiation to become skeletal muscle cells, under different conditions they may undergo milieu-dependent differentiation to manifest other phenotypes. In the context of myoblast implantation into the myocardium, it can be postulated that at least two experimental conditions may affect the differentiation of the implanted cells, thus offering an explanation to the observations made (which are described above).

Confluence Hypothesis

It is proposed that the culture conditions of the satellite cells before implantation may affect their differentiation and phenotype expression after intramyocardial implantation. It has been known for many years that satellite cells in culture will retain their myoblast characteristics and continue to multiply, provided that the cellular density in the culture is kept low. This can be accomplished by repeatedly splitting the culture plates so that the total number of cells can be increased without increasing cell density in each culture plate. However, if this is not done and cellular density in the culture plate is allowed to increase, a point will be reached when the cells will cease to divide, will become confluent, and will differentiate in culture into multinucleated muscle fibers (Fig 2). As stated earlier, the development of skeletal muscle cells is determined by the expression of genes encoding myogenic transcription factors of the MyoD family. Thus, in the in vitro culture conditions, crowding of cells may trigger the expression of these genes.

There are two possible triggering mechanisms associated with cellular overcrowding in the culture. High cellular density would increase cell-to-cell contact, which may signal the cells to fuse and undergo differentiation. Alternately, the cells may be secreting certain signaling molecules to the environment, namely the culture medium, and when these signaling molecules reach a certain level, it could initiate myoblast fusion and the formation of multicellular striated muscle fibers. An experimental study designed to address this question, involving culturing the same density of myoblasts under a different amount of culture media, strongly suggested that the latter mechanism is the likely explanation for this phenomenon. In spite of the same cellular densities in the two plates, the one containing a greater amount of culture media delayed cellular fusion and differentiation.[56]

Our *confluence hypothesis* postulates that if the satellite cells are cultured in vitro before implantation, and if the culture is performed under conditions that allow the cells to cease dividing and to proceed to fuse, the cascade initiated by the MyoD family will continue to drive the differentiating myocytes after implantation to exhibit skeletal myocyte phenotype. In other words, the cells already triggered in vitro to pursue a differentiation pathway toward the skeletal muscle will continue to do so after implantation, and they can no longer be affected by the cardiac milieu they find themselves. On the other hand, satellite cells cultured in vitro in a condition that avoided triggering cell confluence will retain their ability to adapt to the new environment found within the myocardium at the time of implantation. It is also speculated that intermediate conditions between these two extremes may occur that may produce cells that appear mosaic in their phenotype expressions (Fig 7).[55]

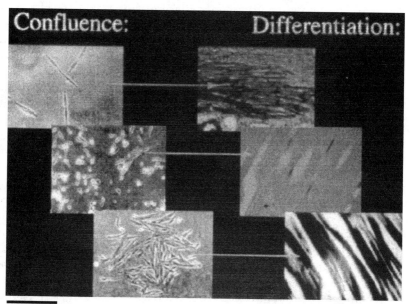

FIGURE 7.
Graphic illustration of the confluence hypothesis. When the satellite cells are cultured under conditions of low cellular density, the cells may maintain their myoblast potential to undergo "milieu-dependent differentiation" on implantation into the myocardium and develop into striated muscle with cardiac phenotype *(upper panel)*. In contrast, satellite cells cultured under high-density conditions may initiate their differentiation programs such that, on implantation into the myocardium, they may grow into striated muscle with skeletal myofiber characteristics *(lower panel)*. With the mixture of these culture conditions, they may differentiate into mosaic striated muscle fibers, exhibiting both cardiac and skeletal muscle fiber phenotypes in the same tissue *(middle panel)*. This hypothesis is advanced to explain varied phenotype outcomes observed with satellite cell implantation into the myocardium and may require further rigorous confirmation.

Community Effects

The science of *topobiology* is to elucidate the mechanisms of how cellular environments may affect their differentiation and phenotypic expressions.[28] The microenvironment surrounding the cells is known to be able to modulate cellular shape, migration, proliferation, and metabolic activities through complex interactions of changes in ECM, cell-to-cell contact, and signaling. Cell membrane receptors and the cytoskeletal system appear to play important roles in the transduction of external signals to intracellular activities. It is postulated that adult skeletal myoblasts implanted into the myocardium may be modulated by this new and unique environment to express some or many phenotypic characteristics of a cardiac myocyte. This community effect could occur through direct cell-to-cell contact or by some signaling molecules, such as certain growth factors or adhesion molecules. A recent study[51] reported that myoblasts implanted into a cryolesion of the heart differentiated into skeletal muscle cells when they were located in the center of the scar tissue, whereas those in the periphery of the scar adjacent to the surviving native myocardium showed ultrastructural morphology similar to immature cardiac myocytes. This suggests that the environmental factor responsible may have to be in close proximity to the implanted cells. Whether this proximity involves cell-to-cell contact or other molecular signals is not clear at this time, and further investigations are needed.

It appears, therefore, that conditions both before and after the cell implantation may affect the outcome in such an experiment. Further elucidation and confirmation of these factors will be most important in obtaining a consistent and reliable outcome if cell implantation is to be considered for therapeutic use.

FUNCTIONAL STUDIES

Another major step required before the clinical application of cardiac cell implantation is the demonstration of the functional contribution of the neomyocardium. Studies in a number of animal models have shown that tissues derived from implanted cells may indeed contribute to the function of the injured heart. It would appear at this time that there may be two mechanisms for such functional effects.

VENTRICULAR REMODELING (SHIELDING) EFFECT

Global ventricular function has been studied using a Langendorff preparation in vitro on rat hearts into which fetal cardiac myocytes was implanted within a myocardial cryolesion.[57] Compared with the control animals in which culture media were injected, the cell-implanted hearts demonstrated better peak systolic pressure and contractility. Histologically, these fetal cardiac myocytes do not appear to have fully differentiated to form mature striated muscle fibers, and no clear connection with the native myocardium was demonstrated. Thus, this study does not indicate that these new myocytes are contracting in synchrony with the native myocardium. Nevertheless, the size of the hearts and of the scar tissue appear to be much smaller than those of the controls, suggesting that the improvement in the global ventricular function observed could be caused by the modulating effect of the implanted tissue in reducing cardiac dilatation resulting from cryoinjury. It has been suggested that the presence of muscle tissue within the scar, regardless of its phenotype, may have a *shielding effect,* reducing the progressive scar expansion and cardiac dilatation seen in the control specimens.

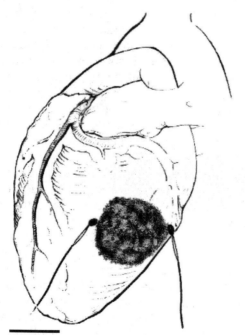

FIGURE 8.
An experimental model to determine the functional contribution of new tissue grown from implanted satellite cells within a cryoinjured left ventricular myocardium. Implanted miniature cylindrical ultrasonic transducers can measure minor axis mid-wall segmental length changes within the region of the cryoinjury with or without cell implantation. The pressure-fiber length loops obtained allow for a load-independent evaluation of changes in regional myocardial function. (Courtesy of Lewis CW, Atkins BZ, Hutcheson KA, et al: A load-independent in vivo model for evaluating therapeutic interventions in injured myocardium. *Am J Physiol* 275:H1834-H1844, 1998. Copyright the American Physiological Society.)

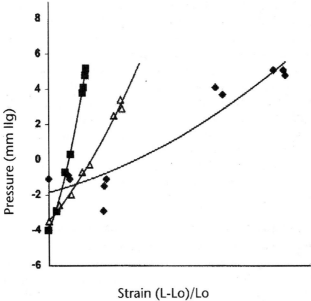

FIGURE 9.

Regional diastolic function obtained using the technique illustrated in Figure 8. Regional relationships relating left ventricular end-diastolic pressure in mmHg with regional myocardial strain (L-Lo)/Lo as an indication of compliance or stiffness, where *L* is end-diastolic segment length and *Lo* is the minimal end-diastolic segment length obtained over the intervention for that animal. A steeper curve indicates increased stiffness or decreased compliance. The shift rightward and the less-steep curve after myoblast engraftment indicated decreased stiffness (i.e., increased compliance) after cellular cardiomyoplasty. (Courtesy of Taylor DA, Atkins BZ, Hungspreugs P, et al: Regenerating functional myocardium: Improved performance after skeletal myoblast transplantation. *Nat Med* 4:929-933, 1998.)

DYNAMIC AUGMENTATION OF VENTRICULAR FUNCTION

The dynamic systolic efficacy of the tissue developed from implanted autologous satellite cells has been shown in a canine coronary occlusion model.[58] In contrast to the hearts that did not receive cell implants, the hearts with implanted cells demonstrated ventricular wall thickening at the sites where the cells were implanted. Similar findings were observed in a cyroinjured model of rabbit hearts,[59] in which changes in the fiber length across the implanted area in the ventricle were plotted against changes in ventricular pressure (Fig 8). The pressure-length loops generated in such animals again indicated that the new muscle fibers developed from implanted cells contributed to the systolic contractile function of the hearts and to improvement in diastolic compliance

(Fig 9).[60] It is not clear from these studies whether such effects were accomplished as the result of the desmosomal junctions developing between the neomyocardium and the native myocardium, allowing for synchronous depolarization of these muscles. An alternate possibility is that, in the absence of such specialized cellular connections, the neomyocardium may still contract in synchrony with the native muscle in response to scar stretching; this stretching is caused by increased systolic pressure, which in turn is generated by the remaining native myocardium. The surgeons are aware that hearts in systolic arrest may respond with a contraction to mechanical stimulation, such as tapping the heart with the surgeon's hand. It is expected that future electrophysiologic studies may dissolve such questions.

FUNCTIONAL IMPLICATIONS OF MUSCLE PHENOTYPES

If, because of certain implant conditions as discussed above, the implanted satellite cells develop into skeletal muscle fibers in the heart, perhaps systolic assist may be achievable only when pacemaker technology is applied to deliver synchronized burst stimulation to the intramyocardial skeletal muscle mass (in a way similar to that used for dynamic cardiomyoplasty). It is possible that skeletal muscle fibers within the scar tissue may still ameliorate cardiac dysfunction by the shielding effect discussed earlier.

Ideally, however, the goal of satellite cell cardiac implantation should be producing neomyocardium tissue that is capable of forming desmosome cell junctions with the native cardiac myocytes. Such junctional structures have indeed been observed at the periphery of the infarct zone, where the tissue grown from implanted cells and the surviving native myocardium tissues come into contact. If this is accomplished, the neomyocardium will become part of the myocardial syncytium, thus achieving the therapeutic goal of regenerating the myocardium to replace damaged myocardial tissue.

FUTURE PERSPECTIVES
CLINICAL TRIALS: POSSIBLE BENEFITS AND RISKS

As mentioned in the introduction, autologous cell implantation has the clinical advantage of not requiring a donor individual, as well as avoiding the need for immunosuppression. These features would be favorable for early clinical trials in patients who may benefit from such therapy. However, before a clinical trial, it would be desirable to elucidate a number of issues that could be important in the ultimate usefulness of such treatments. At this time, it is not known how many satellite cells may be realistically harvested from the patient's own skeletal muscle, nor how much they can be proliferated in vitro by culture. The amount of neomyocardium that could be grown from the known quantity of cells implanted needs to be determined. The choice for the routes of cell implantation may depend on the pathology of the heart, with transmyocardial injection preferable for localized myocardial damage and transcoronary injection more suitable for cardiomyopathies, perhaps. Another obvious question is whether the neomyocardial tissue implanted into the ischemic zone of the heart may spontaneously induce angiogenesis, as is known to occur during organogenesis and oncogenesis, or whether the satellite cells should undergo genetic engineering, such as transfection with vascular endothelial growth factor (VEGF) genes before implantation, while these cells are cultured in vitro. Expression of such VEGF genes after cell implantation may augment blood supply to the new tissue.

FROM IN-VIVO TISSUE ENGINEERING TO ORGANOGENESIS

We started this chapter by pondering how cardiac surgery might look in the next millennium. The in vivo tissue engineering of the heart through regeneration of myocardial tissue with cell implantation would only be the first step of the biological revolution that will finally reach the practice of cardiac surgery. One can imagine not only regenerating the myocardium, but also the cardiac conducting system. Damaged cardiac valves may not be replaced with plastic or animal tissues, but by autologous, in vitro tissue-engineered valves. If we learn how to guide myoblasts to differentiate in the pathway of our choice, perhaps we could consider the dream of applying this *guided differentiation* technique to even more primitive stem cells for cardiac organogenesis, thus enabling a cardiac isograft rather than an allograft. Then the truism that today's science fiction is tomorrow's scientific reality will continue to be realized into the new millennium.

REFERENCES

1. Satava RM: The virtual surgeon. *The Sciences* 38:34-39, 1998.
2. Chiu RCJ: Patient advocate versus societal gate-keeper and the future of high-tech medicine (editorial). *Pacing Clin Electrophysiol* 17:135-137, 1993.
3. Shinoka T, Ma PX, Shum-Tim D, et al: Tissue engineering heart valves: Autologous valve leaflet replacement study in a lamb model. *Circulation* 94:164S-168S, 1996.
4. Zibaitis A, Greentree D, Ma F, et al: Myocardial regeneration with satellite cell implantation. *Transpl Proc* 26:3294, 1994.
5. Soonpaa MH, Koh GY, Klug MG, et al: Formation of nascent intercalated disks between grafted cardiomyocytes and host myocardium. *Science* 264:98-101, 1994.

6. Robinson SW, Cho PW, Levitsky HI, et al: Arterial delivery of genetically labelled skeletal myoblasts to the murine heart: Long-term survival and phenotypic modification of implanted myoblasts. *Cell Transpl* 5:77-91, 1996.

7. Marelli D, Desrosiers C, El-Alfy M, et al: Cell transplantation for myocardial repair: An experimental approach. *Cell Transplant* 1:383-390, 1992.

8. Li RK, Yau TM, Sakai T, et al: Cell therapy to repair broken hearts. *Can J Cardiol* 14:735-744, 1998.

9. Kao RL, Chiu RCJ (eds): *Cellular Cardiomyoplasty: Cellular Implantation for Myocardial Replacement.* Austin, Tex, RG Landes, 1997.

10. Tam SKC, Gu W, Mahdavi V, et al: Cardiac myocyte terminal differentiation: Potential for cardiac regeneration. *Ann NY Acad Sci* 752:72-79, 1995.

11. Zak R: Development and proliferation capacity of cardiac muscle cells. *Circ Res* 35:17S-26S, 1974.

12. Li F, Wang X, Capasso JM, et al: Rapid transition of cardiac myocytes from hyperplasia to hypertrophy during postnatal development. *J Mol Cell Cardiol* 28:1737-1746, 1996.

13. Schultz E: Fine structure of satellite cells in growing skeletal muscle. *Am J Anat* 147:49-70, 1976.

14. Mauro A: Satellite cells of skeletal muscle fibres. *J Biophys Biochem Cytol* 9:493-495, 1961.

15. Lipton BH, Schultz E: Developmental fate of skeletal muscle satellite cells. *Science* 205:1292-1294, 1979.

16. Nag AC, Carey TR, Cheng M: DNA synthesis in rat heart cells after injury and the regeneration of myocardia. *Tissue Cell* 15:597-613, 1983.

17. Almeddine HS, Dehaupas M, Fardeau M: Regeneration of skeletal muscle fibres from autologous satellite cells multiplied in vitro: An experimental model for testing cultured cell myogenicity. *Muscle Nerve* 12:544-555, 1989.

18. Carlson BM: The generation of skeletal muscle: A review. *Am J Anat* 137:119, 1973.

19. Schmalbruch H, Hellhammer U: The number of satellite cells in normal human muscle. *Anat Rec* 185:279-288, 1976.

20. Schultz E, Jaryszak DL, Valliere CB: Response of satellite cells to focal skeletal muscle injury. *Muscle Nerve* 8:217-222, 1985.

21. Matsuda R, Spector DH, Strohman RC: Regenerating adult chicken skeletal muscle and satellite cell cultures express embryonic patterns of myosin and tropomyosin isoforms. *Dev Biol* 100:478-488, 1983.

22. Jones P: In vitro comparison of embryonic myoblasts and myogenic cells isolated from regenerating adult rat skeletal muscle. *Exp Cell Res* 139:401-404, 1982.

23. Watt DJ, Morgan TE, Clifford MA, et al: The movement of muscle precursor cells between adjacent regenerating muscle in the mouse. *Anat Embryol* 175:527-536, 1987.

24. Yaffe D, Feldman M: The formation of hybrid multinucleated muscle fibres from myoblasts of different genetic origin. *Dev Biol* 11:300-317, 1965.

25. Schultz E, Albright DJ, Jaryszak DL, et al: Survival of satellite cells in whole muscle transplants. *Anat Rec* 222:12-17, 1988.
26. Eguchi G, Kodama R: Transdifferentiation. *Curr Opin Cell Biol* 5:1023-1028, 1993.
27. Furnary AP, Jessup M, Moreira LFP: Multicenter trial of dynamic cardiomyoplasty for chronic heart failure. *J Am Coll Cardiol* 28:1175-1180, 1996.
28. Edelman GM: *Topobiology: An Introduction to Molecular Embryology.* New York, Harper-Collins, 1988.
29. Katagiri T, Yamaguchi A, Komaki M, et al: Bone morphogenetic protein-2 converts the differentiation pathway of C2C12 myoblasts into the osteoblast lineage. *J Cell Biol* 127:1755-1766, 1994.
30. Cossu G, Kelly R, Di Donna S, et al: Myoblast differentiation during mammalian somitogenesis is dependent upon a community effect. *Proc Natl Acad Sci U S A* 92:2254-2258, 1995.
31. Osdoby P, Caplan AI: Characterization of bone-specific alkaline phosphatase in cultures of chick limb mesenchymal cells. *Dev Biol* 86:136-146, 1981.
32. Field LJ: Atrial natriuretic factor-SV40 T antigen transgenes produce tumors and cardiac arrhythmias in mice. *Science* 239:1029-1033, 1988.
33. Weintraub H, Davis R, Tapscott S, et al: The myoD gene family: Nodal point during specification of the muscle cell lineage. *Science* 251:761-766, 1991.
34. Sartorelli V, Hong NA, Bishopric NH, et al: Myocardial activation of the human cardiac α-actin promoter by helix-loop-helix proteins. *Proc Natl Acad Sci U S A* 89:4047-4051, 1992.
35. Navankasattussas S, Zhu H, Garcia AV, et al: A ubiquitous factor (HF-1a) and a distinct muscle factor (HF-lb/MEF2) form an E-box–independent pathway for cardiac muscle gene expression. *Mol Cell Biol* 12:1469-1679, 1991.
36. Chen G, Birnbaum RS, Yablonka-Reuveni Z, et al: Separation of mouse crushed muscle extract into distinct mitogenic activities by heparin affinity chromatography. *J Cell Physiol* 160:563-572, 1994.
37. Kardami E, Fandrich RR: Basic fibroblast growth factor in atria and ventricles of the vertebrate heart. *J Cell Biol* 109:1865-1875, 1989.
38. Engelmann GL, Dionne CA, Jaye MC: Acidic fibroblast growth factor and heart development: Role in myocyte proliferation and capillary angiogenesis. *Circ Res* 72:7-19, 1993.
39. Olson EN, Sternberg E, Hu JS, et al: Regulation of myogenic differentiation by type beta transforming factor. *J Cell Biol* 103:1799-1805, 1986.
40. MacLellan WR, Brand T, Schneider MD: Transforming growth factor-β in cardiac ontogeny and adaptation. *Circ Res* 73:783-791, 1993.
41. Villarreal FJ, Dillmann WH: Cardiac hypertrophy–induced changes in mRNA levels for TGF-beta 1, fibronectin, and collagen. *Am J Physiol* 262:H1861-H1866, 1992.
42. Coleman ME, DeMayo F, Yin KC, et al: Myogenic vector expression of insulin-like growth factor I stimulates muscle cell differentiation and myofiber hypertrophy in transgenic mice. *J Biol Chem* 270:12109-12116, 1995.

43. Rosenthal SM, Brown EJ: Mechanisms of insulin-like growth factor (IGF)-II–induced IGF-I receptor down-regulation in BC3H-1 muscle cells. *J Endocrinol* 141:69-74, 1994.
44. Griffith CM, Sanders EJ: Effects of extracellular matrix components on the differentiation of chick embryo tail bud mesenchyme in culture. *Differentiation* 47:61-68, 1991.
45. Iruela-Arispe ML, Sage EH: Expression of type VIII collagen during morphogenesis of the chicken and mouse heart. *Dev Biol* 144:107-118, 1991.
46. Mosher DF: Physiology of fibronectin. *Ann Rev Med* 35:561-575, 1984.
47. Enomoto MI, Boettiger D, Menko AS: Alpha 5 integrin is a critical component of adhesion plaques in myogenesis. *Dev Biol* 155:180-197, 1993.
48. Peck D, Walsh FS: Differential effects of over-expressed neural cell adhesion molecule isoforms on myoblast fusion. *J Cell Biol* 123:1587-1595, 1993.
49. Moore R, Walsh FS: The cell adhesion molecule M-cadherin is specifically expressed in developing and regenerating, but not denervated skeletal muscle. *Development* 117:1409-1420, 1993.
50. Chiu RC-J, Zibaitis A, Kao RL: Cellular cardiomyoplasty: Myocardial regeneration with satellite cell implantation. *Ann Thorac Surg* 60:12-18, 1995.
51. Atkins BZ, Lewis CW, Kraus WE, et al: Intracardiac transplantation of skeletal myoblasts yields two populations of striated cells in situ. *Ann Thorac Surg* 67:124-129, 1999.
52. Dorfman J, Duong M, Zibaitis A, et al: Myocardial tissue engineering with autologous myoblast implantation. *J Thorac Cardiovasc Surg* 116:744-751, 1998.
53. Greentree D, Marelli D, Ma F, et al: Labelling techniques in satellite cell transplantation. *Transplant Proc* 26:3357, 1994.
54. Taylor DA, Silvestry SC, Bishop SP, et al: Delivery of primary autologous skeletal myoblasts into rabbit heart by coronary infusion: A potential approach to myocardial repair. *Proc Assoc Am Physicians* 109:245-253, 1997.
55. Zibaitis A, Ma F, Duong M, et al: Cellular cardiomyoplasty: Results and possibilities for the future. *Cardiovasc Eng* 1:55-59, 1996.
56. Konigsberg IR, Buckley PA: Regulation of the cell cycle in myogenesis by cell medium interaction, in J Lash, JR Whittaker (eds): *Concepts of Development*. Stamford, Conn, Sinauer, 1974, pp 179-193.
57. Li RK, Jia Z-Q, Weisel RD, et al: Cardiomyocyte transplantation improves heart function. *Ann Thorac Surg* 62:654-661, 1996.
58. Kao RL, Davis J, Kao GW, et al: Myocardial regeneration improves heart function. *FASEB J* 12:A5651, 1998.
59. Lewis CW, Atkins BZ, Hutcheson KA, et al: A load-independent in vivo model for evaluating therapeutic interventions in injured myocardium. *Am J Physiol* 275:H1834-H1844, 1998.
60. Taylor DA, Atkins BZ, Hungspreugs P, et al: Regenerating functional myocardium: Improved performance after skeletal myoblast transplantation. *Nat Med* 4:929-933, 1998.

CHAPTER 5

The Radial Artery as a Graft for Coronary Revascularization: Techniques and Follow-up

James Tatoulis, M.B.B.S., F.R.A.C.S.
Senior Academic Associate, University of Melbourne; Director of Cardiac Surgery, Royal Melbourne Hospital, Melbourne, Victoria, Australia

Brian F. Buxton, M.B.M.S., F.R.A.C.S., F.R.C.S.
Professor of Cardiac Surgery, University of Melbourne; Director of Cardiac Surgery, Austin and Repatriation Medical Centre, Melbourne, Victoria, Australia

John A. Fuller, M.B.B.S., F.R.A.C.P., F.R.C.P.(Edin)
Chief of Perfusion, Epworth Hospital, Melbourne, Victoria, Australia

Alistair G. Royse, M.B.B.S., F.R.A.C.S.
Surgical Associate and Examiner, University of Melbourne; Cardiothoracic Surgeon, Royal Melbourne Hospital, Melbourne, Victoria, Australia

The first use of the radial artery (RA) as an aortocoronary bypass graft was reported in 1973 by Carpentier et al.,[1] who used 40 RA grafts in 30 patients. RA spasm encountered during harvesting was managed with mechanical dilation. The short-term results were good, with no mortality, only a 10% recurrence of angina and a greater than 90% early patency, and only 1 (3%) early reoperation. However, within 2 years it became apparent that the medium-term results were extremely disappointing, with 32% of the grafts occluded and an additional significant proportion with severe generalized stenosis,[2] and hence, the use of the RA graft was abandoned. Traumatic harvesting and mechanical dilation were thought to have caused severe endothelial injury, hyperplasia, and spasm.[3] Seventeen years later (1992), Acar[4] from Carpentier's group revived the use of the RA after unexpected good long-term results from the early cohort of patients operated on before 1973. A number of grafts, angiographically demonstrated to be "occluded" in 1973, were found to be fully patent, smooth, and without any sign of intimal disease 15 to 18 years later.

During a 3-year period from 1989 to 1992, Acar et al.[4] used 122 RAs in 104 patients, in conjunction with internal thoracic arteries (ITAs; 148 grafts) and saphenous veins (24 grafts). All 56 RA grafts studied early were patent, and 29 (93.5%) of 31 RA grafts studied at 9.2 months were patent. This vast improvement in angiographic results occurred because of improved harvesting techniques (mobilizing the artery as a pedicle with its venae comitantes), antispasm management with papaverine, temporary storage in a blood-papaverine solution, use of intravenous diltiazem perioperatively as an antispasmodic, and long-term aspirin and diltiazem therapy.

The landmark report of Acar et al. stimulated many surgeons to explore the use of the RA in coronary surgery, particularly as the second graft of choice after the ITA. Dietl et al.,[5] Brodman et al.,[6] Fremes et al.,[7] Calafiore et al.,[8] and Tatoulis et al.[9] have all recorded significant experiences with the use of the RA, with excellent clinical and early angiographic results.

The challenge for cardiac surgeons is to document the long-term results achieved by use of the RA as a conduit in coronary bypass surgery, and to explore and establish its optimum mode of use in combination with other conduits available, particularly the ITA.

RATIONALE FOR USE OF RA AS A CORONARY BYPASS GRAFT

The ITAs (especially the pedicled left ITA [LITA]) are indisputably the best grafts in coronary revascularization in terms of long-term patency, freedom from recurrent angina, and cardiac events.[10] The right ITA (RITA) used either as a pedicled or as a free graft achieves patency rates similar but usually inferior to the pedicled LITA.[11] Extended arterial revascularization with ITA grafts has been achieved by the use of bilateral ITA grafts,[11,12] the use of "T" or "Y" grafts,[13] and of multiple sequential anastomoses.[12] Frequently, however, the ITA grafts may not reach distally in the inferior circumflex or posterior descending artery (PDA) distribution (even as a free graft), especially if the heart is large.

Other arterial grafts have had limited use because only a short length is available (inferior epigastric artery), or concerns exist regarding additional abdominal surgery and conduit spasm (right gastroepiploic artery). Additionally, the presence of insulin-dependent diabetes and severe pulmonary disease has limited the widespread use of bilateral ITA grafts.[14]

The long-term clinical results and patencies for vein grafts have been disappointing, with reports of less than 50% patency at 10 years, and intraluminal disease found in those grafts that were patent. In all angiographic studies, the patency rate for arterial grafts is consistently higher than that for vein grafts, at any given point after coronary surgery.[15]

The ease of procurement and the encouraging recent results in the use of RA grafts make them an attractive coronary conduit to supplement the use of ITAs. The RA is superficial, readily accessible, and can be harvested with minimal trauma to the conduit itself and to the surrounding structures of the forearm. There are potentially two RA conduits available in each patient. Up to 22 cm of length may be available (per RA conduit), allowing uncompromised deployment distally beyond any stenosis or atheromatous plaque. The nature and texture of the RA conduit allow facile handling and the creation of multiple sequential anastomoses if required. The RA conduit is an appropriate size for the coronary arteries, being a little larger, and it can be harvested simultaneously with sternotomy and harvesting of the LITA, allowing for an efficient conduct of the prebypass phase of the operation.[9,16]

The ready availability, ease of procurement of the RA, and its potential for better long-term patency than that for vein grafts has made it, in our practice, a very attractive alternative as the second coronary graft conduit (after the ITAs). When appropriate, we further extended this concept using bilateral RA grafts particularly to achieve improved long-term myocardial perfusion to the inferior and inferolateral aspect of the left ventricle. RA use is additionally indicated for patients in whom saphenous veins have been stripped or used for vascular procedures, for patients undergoing reoperation for coronary artery disease, for patients who have leg infections, and for patients with severe obstructive airways disease, obesity, or insulin-dependent diabetes, which precludes the use of bilateral ITA grafts.

ANATOMY OF RA

An excellent account of the surgical anatomy of the RA has been published by Reyes et al.[17]

COURSE OF RA

The RA branches from the brachial artery proximal to the biceps tendon. It enters the forearm just medial to the biceps tendon and runs deep to the brachioradialis muscle in loose areolar tissue and runs in a groove between the bulk of the brachioradialis laterally and the pronator teres and flexor carpi radialis medially. In the distal third of the forearm, the RA becomes superficial, covered only by skin and subcutaneous and fascial tissue, and at the wrist the RA is located between the brachioradialis tendon laterally and the flexor carpi radialis tendon medially.

BRANCHES FROM PROXIMAL TO DISTAL

The first branch is a recurrent branch originating soon after the origin of the RA and running proximally and laterally. Usually this vessel would be preserved. In the proximal third of the forearm, there are one or two larger branches (0.2-0.5 mm) originating from the deep surface of the RA and running to the brachioradialis muscle directly, and also to the interosseous space. There are usually five to seven additional branches in the upper two thirds of the forearm predominantly rising from the deep aspect of the artery, and can be well defined in the loose areolar tissue.

As the artery progresses distally, the branches become more frequent, smaller, shorter, and more delicate, and are placed deep, on either side of the RA and also occasionally on the superficial aspect. At its terminal end, the RA supplies branches to the superficial and eventually deep palmar arches. These branches are usually beyond the wrist joint; however, occasionally the superficial palmar arch branch may arise several centimeters above the wrist joint.

VEINS AND ORIENTATION

The RA is surrounded by satellite veins (venae comitantes) that accompany the artery from distal to proximal and contribute bridging branches to each other along the course of the RA, and to a large plexus of veins just distal to the origin of the RA from the brachial.

There is a 90-degree rotation of the RA vascular pedicle, commencing in a plane parallel to the wrist distally, to a 90-degree medial rotation at the elbow.

NERVES

The lateral cutaneous nerve of the forearm (lateral antebrachial cutaneous nerve) is superficial to and runs near the medial border of the brachioradialis. It should be avoided by placing the skin incision medial to the brachioradialis edge.

The superficial radial nerve (SRN) supplies the sensory function to the lateral aspect of the thumb and dorsum of the hand. The SRN runs parallel and lateral to the RA under cover of the brachioradialis in the proximal two thirds of the forearm. Distally the nerve passes under the tendon of the brachioradialis to supply the distal forearm and hand. Accidental trauma (traction, bruising) to the SRN will invariably cause sensory abnormalities in the lateral aspect of the thumb and dorsum of the hand.

ANATOMICAL VARIATIONS

The most common variation is a high origin of the RA (high bifurcation of the brachial artery), occurring in up to 2% of upper limbs. In 1% of limbs, a small but significant branch of the RA runs superficial to the brachioradialis muscle, with the normal vessel being correctly placed. The distal termination of the RA can be variable, with a relatively high branch to the superficial palmar arch or a totally absent superficial arch; under these circumstances, the RA is the dominant vascular supply of the hand.[18,19]

HISTOLOGY

The RA has a relatively thin intima. The internal elastic lamina is well developed but fenestrated. The media is the dominant layer, is highly muscular, and maybe a significant reason for the predisposition of the vessel to spasm. The muscular media is bounded by the external elastic lamina, which is thicker than the internal one and similarly fenestrated. The adventitia is of modest thickness, being 50% to 100% of the thickness of the muscular media. The adventitia has a significant number of vasa vasora.

Generally the thickness of the RA wall is 500 μm (0.5 mm) (by comparison with the ITA average of 200 μm). The ratio of wall thickness to internal diameter of the proximal RA is less than at the distal end. Additionally, the RA is more likely to have intimal thickening with lipid deposition, both intracellular and extracellular, in comparison with the ITA. Brodman et al.[20] found 72% of RAs had normal or minimal intimal changes but 28% had significant atherosclerotic intimal changes in 106 specimens. By comparison, only 6% of 64 ITAs had significant intimal atherosclerotic changes. The presence of diabetes, peripheral vascular disease, and male gender correlated with an increase in RA pathology. Our experience has been similar, with 6 of 24 RA specimens examined consecutively having significant lipid and atheromatous changes in the intima.[21] The mean distal RA diameter (2.24 ± 0.37 mm) was significantly larger than that of an ITA (2.02 ± 0.23 mm) in the same patient. This was true proximally as well.

PHARMACOLOGY

The RA is extremely prone to spasm on mechanical or other stimulation (cold), with a potent vasoconstrictive response that is stronger than that of the ITA. Chardigny et al.[22] showed that the RA and gastroepiploic arteries presented a higher contraction force than the ITA. This has been corroborated by He and Yang,[23] and in our own laboratory where we found the maximal contractile response of the RA to vasoconstrictors (norepinephrine, 5-hydroxytryptamine, thromboxane A_2, and endothelin-1) was twice that of the ITA.[24]

The potential reactivity of the muscular layer of the RA, particularly at the distal end where the lumen is smaller and the ratio of media to internal diameter greater, is of extreme significance, requiring strategies to overcome induced spasm in the short term, medium term, and long term.

GENERAL PHILOSOPHY AND SURGICAL STRATEGY

Our philosophy has been to regard the RA as the graft of second choice after the ITAs. The disappointing results of saphenous vein grafts has made the concept of total arterial revascularization (TAR) extremely attractive and potentially crucial for improved long-term results.

Because the RA is readily available and the recent (though limited) experience has been favorable, we have undertaken a strategy of the predominant use of one or two ITA grafts, together with one or two RA grafts, to achieve TAR.

ASSESSMENT OF ADEQUACY OF ULNAR ARTERY COLLATERAL CIRCULATION TO THE HAND (MODIFIED ALLEN'S TEST)

Before harvesting the RA, the adequacy of the ulnar artery collateral circulation must be established. We have routinely used the modified Allen's test. Both radial and ulnar arteries are compressed just above the wrist for 30 seconds, during which time the hand is rendered ischemic by strong clenching of the fist and subsequent slow relaxation, repeated three times. The ulnar artery is released, and the hyperemic response in the hand extending to the thenar eminence and the thumb is observed. A rapid response is deemed to have occurred if it was within 5 seconds, and a satisfactory response if within 10 seconds, both indicating satisfactory ulnar collaterals and nondominance of the RA. A response beyond 10 seconds is deemed unsatisfactory, and the RA is not used. In general, when the ulnar collateral circulation is inadequate in one hand, it is also inadequate in the other hand. In our institution, 2% of patients had a dominant RA that was not harvested.[9]

A total of 382 consecutive patients in our institution were evaluated both preoperatively and postoperatively in detail with regard to possible hand and finger ischemia after RA harvest at 3, 6, and 12 months (Table 1). Ischemic symptoms developed in only

TABLE 1.

Relationship Between Ulnar Collateral Supply to the Hand and Hand Ischemia in 380 Patients

	Ulnar Collateral Time (Modified Allen's Test)		
	<5 sec	**6-10 sec**	**>10 sec**
No. of patients	306	72	Radial not used
Ischemic symptoms	0	2 (3%)	

2 patients, both of whom had a chronic collagen disease (scleroderma), as well as ulnar collateral reaction times of 6 to 10 seconds. The first patient had Raynaud's phenomenon in cold weather that responded well to long-term calcium antagonists. The other had ischemia at the tip of the index finger requiring amputation of the distal 1 cm. There were no other ischemic problems, and pulse plethysmography showed no difference in the waveforms and oxygen saturations by pulse oximetry (mean, 97.8% ± 0.5%) from preoperative values. Others have advocated Doppler testing of the RA,[25] noninvasive oximetric plethysmography,[16] or the additional use of an intraoperative Allen's test once the RA has been mobilized but before it is transected,[5] all of which are reliable and effective assessments.

OPERATIVE TECHNIQUE
PREPARATION AND DRAPING
The forearms are marked preoperatively for RA harvest to ensure awareness and prevention of inadvertent cannulation of the RA or forearm veins by the anesthetist. The patient is prepared and draped as for standard coronary artery bypass grafting (CABG). The arms are prepared and draped at the same time, after they have been abducted 70 to 80 degrees from the torso and placed on arm boards with specifically shaped soft jelly-like contours to maintain position.

LITA and RA
If only one RA is required, the left RA is usually harvested, simultaneously with the sternotomy and harvesting of the LITA. This is the most common scenario.

Bilateral ITAs and a Single RA
Initially, the procedure would be as described above. In addition, once the left RA is harvested, the left forearm is closed, dressed,

bandaged, and placed beside the torso; an additional sterile drape is placed, and the RITA is then harvested.

LITA and Bilateral RAs

Both RAs are harvested by two independent operators simultaneously. The wounds are closed, dressed and bandaged, the arms are placed by the side of the torso, additional drapes are placed, and the sternal part of the operation commences.

Unusual Circumstances

Occasionally, the right RA is preferred (patient is left-handed, better ulnar collateral circulation, or the left RA has been previously cannulated), or the RITA is required (as in a redo). The initial part of the operation proceeds in a mirror image of scenario 1 (LITA and left RA).

ANESTHETIC PREPARATION

The arterial line is placed in the opposite RA, or in the femoral artery (if bilateral RAs are used). A Swan-Ganz catheter is placed via the right internal jugular vein. Additional venous catheters are placed by a separate internal jugular vein puncture, external jugular vein, or the cephalic vein in the upper arm. An oximeter is placed on the earlobe.

HARVESTING THE RA

An incision with a slight medial curve is made from a point 2 cm proximal to the styloid process of the radius immediately over the RA and proximal to the major skin crease of the wrist, running to a point 2 cm distal to the elbow crease and 1 cm medial to the biceps tendon (Fig 1). The medial curve of the incision allows the operator to avoid the superficial cutaneous nerve of the forearm,

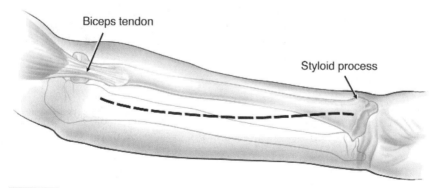

FIGURE 1.
Skin incision for harvesting the left radial artery.

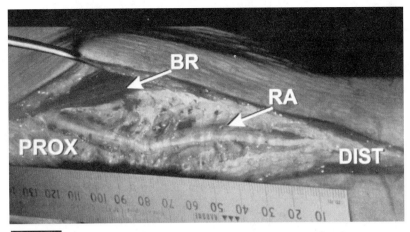

FIGURE 2.
Operative photograph of the left radial artery (*RA*) showing its uniform size and its relationship to the brachioradialis (*BR*). *Abbreviations: PROX,* proximal; *DIST,* distal.

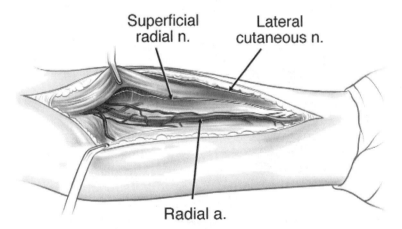

FIGURE 3.
Diagrammatic representation of the left radial artery (*a.*) and its relationship to the superficial radial nerve (*n.*), the brachioradialis, and the lateral cutaneous nerve of the forearm.

and allows access to the medial border of the brachioradialis muscle. The subcutaneous tissues and superficial veins are divided using diathermy. The deep fascia of the forearm is well defined but translucent, and is incised directly over the RA to allow immediate exposure of the RA pedicle and clear identification of the artery and vein branches, particularly on the lateral and deep aspects of the RA (Figs 2 and 3). The smaller branches are clipped on the RA side and divided with diathermy on the other (Fig 4).

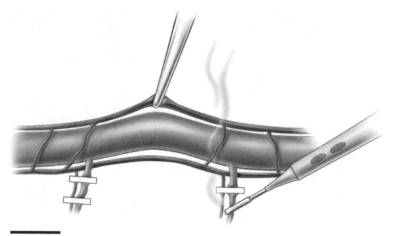

FIGURE 4.

Harvesting the radial artery using a minimal touch technique, to avoid injury to the radial artery; and technique of securing radial artery branches.

The larger branches are divided between small titanium vascular clips. Usually it is a progressive dissection from the distal to proximal. As the RA passes deep and medial to the brachioradialis, this space is opened up by lateral retraction on the brachioradialis with a self-retaining retractor. The tissues here are looser with fewer branches that predominantly pass deep into the brachioradialis or into the interosseous plane. The dissection is performed with an emphasis on minimal touch and minimal diathermy.

When most of the RA has been mobilized, a soft vascular clamp can be placed on the RA pedicle and the retrograde pulsation noted.[5] At the distal end, the satellite veins are separately clipped and divided, and then the RA is divided after securing the distal stump with two medium-sized vascular clips. Retrograde pulsation is usually seen in the distal stump.

Using a bulb-ended vascular 1-mm cannula, 5 mL of 1% papaverine in heparinized blood is placed intraluminally in the RA, and the distal end of the RA is clipped, allowing it to pulsate against the occluded end. The residual proximal branches are secured while the RA is dilating. The proximal end of the dissection is marked by a prominent plexus of veins on the medial aspect of the RA, and also by the recurrent RA branch. Again, the satellite veins are individually secured and divided, and the proximal RA is divided after placement of two medium titanium vascular clips, with at least a 3-mm cuff beyond (Fig 5). The RA is examined, the distal and proximal ends are fashioned for anastomosis, and the conduit is then stored in a 1% papaverine solution of

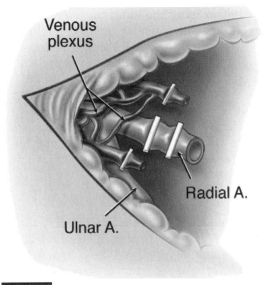

FIGURE 5.
Method of securing the proximal end of the radial artery (*A.*). The venous plexus distal to the brachial artery bifurcation is shown.

heparinized arterial blood, at room temperature, until it is used (20-60 minutes, depending on the procedure).

If the desired length of the RA is known, then the more proximal part of the RA is harvested, leaving the distal smaller portion of the RA in situ with its large number of branches, thus reducing the degree of distal harvesting and leaving more anastomotic connections around the wrist. Additionally, large proximal interosseous or muscular branches are preserved if it is known that the length of the graft would not be compromised.

The SRN usually runs lateral to the RA pedicle and normally is not seen. Care is required not to damage this important sensory nerve.

The vast majority of RA dissection is by a combination of sharp (scissor) dissection and diathermy. However, the Harmonic Scalpel (Ultracision Inc., Smithfield, RI) with an ultrasonic oscillating straight probe at 55 kHz was used for a small minority of cases, with a satisfactory result.

Once the RA is harvested, hemostasis is checked, the subcutaneous layer is closed with a continuous absorbable suture, the skin is closed with a continuous absorbable monofilament subcuticular suture, dressings are placed, and a crepe bandage is applied with firm pressure. The arm is then placed by the side of the torso, and a large new drape is used to cover the side of the patient and the arm.

Because the vast majority of the branches are on the deep side of the RA, the superficial side is usually more favorable if sequential anastomoses are to be constructed. We also take care to avoid diathermy close to the tendons of the brachioradialis and flexor carpi radialis to avoid devascularization of those areas.

The 1% papaverine-blood solution with which the RA is treated, and in which it is stored, must be adequately heparinized to avoid clots within the RA lumen. The heparin concentration is 5 U/mL of blood achieved by adding 10 mL of arterial blood to 10 mL of heparinized Ringer's lactate solution (1,000 U of heparin in 100 mL of Ringer's lactate solution).

OPERATIVE PROCEDURE

The sternal/ITA/cardiac part of the procedure proceeds either simultaneously with the left RA harvest or after bilateral RA harvest. One or two ITAs are procured as required, and the patient is heparinized with 3 mg (300 U) of heparin per kilogram of body weight. Ascending aorta (under epiaortic echocardiographic guidance), right atrial, and coronary sinus cannulas are placed. Cardiopulmonary bypass is conducted at 33°C to 34°C with flows of 2.5 L/min/m^2, and mean arterial pressure is maintained at 80 mm Hg.

Myocardial protection is with an initial dose of antegrade hyperkalemic aspartate-enriched blood cardioplegia at 20°C (700 mL), and an additional 300 mL of retrograde cardioplegia. The septal myocardial temperature is kept at 20°C to 25°C. Further 300-mL doses of retrograde cardioplegia are given after the completion of each anastomosis (distal or proximal), and a final dose of warm aspartate-enriched retrograde cardioplegia is given after completion of the last anastomosis. All anastomoses (distal and proximal) are constructed during a single period of aortic cross-clamping. If an LITA/RA "Y" graft is to be constructed, this is performed before cannulation.

SURGICAL STRATEGIES FOR GRAFTING: USE OF RA

The LITA is routinely anastomosed to the left anterior descending (LAD) artery. If a diagonal artery is to be grafted, then this is achieved by a side-to-side LITA to diagonal anastomosis, in addition to the LITA to the LAD. If the diagonal is laterally placed or high (intermediate), a separate RITA graft is placed, or a short "Y" limb of distal ITA or RA is created from the proximal LITA.

DOUBLE-VESSEL DISEASE

If the patient is younger than 65 years old, the RITA is used as a pedicled graft to the proximal circumflex, or as a free graft to the distal circumflex or posterior descending branch (PDA) of the right coronary artery (RCA). For older patients, the RA is used to the circumflex (single or sequential) or to the PDA.

TRIPLE-VESSEL DISEASE
In patients younger than 65 years, two ITAs are used if possible and the RA is used to revascularize to the most distal vessel (left ventricular [LV] branch of the right or an inferior circumflex marginal). In patients older than 65 years, one RA is anastomosed to the circumflex system (single or sequential) and the second RA is used to revascularize the distal right coronary system (PDA or LV branch).

"Y" GRAFT
An LITA/RA "Y" graft is used to save conduit or if there is insufficient RA length to reach in the inferior aspect of the heart from the aorta, particularly when there is an excellent lie for the graft between multiple sequential circumflex and distal right coronary anastomoses. The use of the RA allows uncompromised coronary grafting, with performance of the distal anastomosis beyond any lesion or atheromatous plaque.

DISTAL ANASTOMOSIS
All the distal radial to coronary artery anastomoses are constructed with continuous 7-0 or 8-0 polypropylene suture on a small (6-mm) needle. The tissues of the pedicle are loosely secured on either side of each anastomosis with interrupted 6-0 polypropylene suture to ensure correct orientation and prevent kinking.

SIDE-TO-SIDE (SEQUENTIAL ANASTOMOSIS)
If anastomosed to a high marginal or intermediate vessel, the RA is angled at 30 to 45 degrees across the coronary. The angulation of the side-to-side anastomosis to a midmarginal vessel depends on the lie that is required for the RA to run smoothly to the distal end-to-side anastomosis. As much as possible, the anastomoses are constructed in a parallel (0-degree) or up to a 30-degree angulation. Generally, the proximal and midmarginal vessels are grafted toward the base of the heart, and the most distal (end-to-side) anastomosis is constructed farther away from the atrioventricular groove (Fig 6). The sequential anastomosis closest to the aorta is constructed first and so on.

DISTAL END-TO-SIDE ANASTOMOSIS
A distal end-to-side anastomosis is constructed in a parallel fashion if possible, or at most at a 30-degree angle to ensure that the graft does not kink at its distal point. Additional interrupted sutures are placed along the course of graft between the pedicle and epicardium

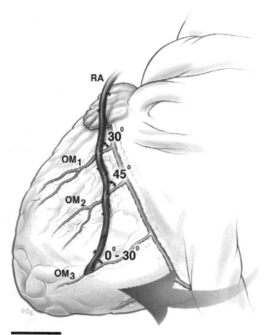

FIGURE 6.
Lie of a sequential radial artery (*RA*) graft with side-to-side anastomosis to the first obtuse marginal artery (*OM₁*), second obtuse marginal artery (*OM₂*), and terminating as an end-to-side anastomosis to the inferior or third obtuse marginal artery (*OM₃*).

to maintain the desired lie. The distance between sequential anastomoses is judged by placing traction in opposite directions between the two coronary vessels in the arrested flaccid heart.

Occasionally if proximal wall disease necessitates sequential grafting distally in the midmarginal artery, the last end-to-side anastomosis can be placed retrogradely on to the most distal vessel. An alternate strategy is to construct a composite RA "Y" graft with a short limb to the proximal marginal (Fig 7). The RA does not kink, and extra length between anastomoses can be well accommodated.

RA GRAFTING TO DISTAL RCA DISTRIBUTION

If a single RA graft is placed to the LV branch of the RA or distal circumflex, it is constructed in a parallel fashion and brought up to the right side of the aorta behind the inferior vena cava (IVC) after incising the pericardial reflection behind the IVC, between the IVC and the inferior pulmonary veins. An isolated RA graft to the PDA is brought anterior to the IVC either following the atrioventricular groove or around the lateral wall of right atrium.

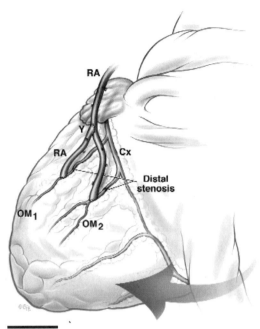

FIGURE 7.
The first circumflex marginal (*OM₁*) has a distal stenosis. The second circumflex marginal (*OM₂*) bifurcates proximally. This anatomical situation is difficult for a sequential grafting technique. It is addressed by a composite radial artery (*RA*) "Y" graft with a short proximal limb end-to-side to the parent RA then placed end-to-side to the coronary vessel. *Abbreviation: Cx,* circumflex.

A sequential graft to the distal right system is constructed by creating the distal end-to-side anastomosis to the LV branch of the RCA first, with an angulation of 30 to 45 degrees, and a side-to-side anastomosis to the PDA angulated at 0 to 90 degrees, depending on the position of the PDA anastomosis. In this instance, care should be taken to ensure that there is a satisfactory RA length to reach the LV branch via the PDA, without undue tension. Any potential shortfall in length should be immediately corrected by end-to-end extension using either a segment of the other RA graft, a short segment of saphenous vein, or proximal attachment to the in situ RITA on the chest wall, with deliberate occlusion of the distal segment of the intact in situ RITA.

PROXIMAL ANASTOMOSES

The proximal anastomosis is usually constructed on to the ascending thoracic aorta, avoiding areas of plaque. A 3.5-mm punch is used to create an opening of appropriate size and shape. The proximal end of the RA is usually of excellent size (3.5-mm diameter), and the wall is easy to handle. A continuous 7-0 polypropylene suture on a larger (9-mm) needle is used if the aorta is normal, or 6-0 polypropylene suture is used with a 12-mm needle if the aorta is slightly thickened. In redo coronary operations, a nonatheromatous proximal vein hood is used for the proximal anastomotic point.

The LITA is frequently used (464 patients) for the proximal anastomosis, either as a deliberate strategy (conduit preservation and/or use of pedicled graft) for additional length, or when the aorta is atheromatous. Rarely, another graft or a pericardial patch on the aorta is used as the site of the proximal anastomosis.

FURTHER INTRAOPERATIVE AND POSTOPERATIVE MANAGEMENT
PROPHYLAXIS AGAINST CONDUIT SPASM

Intravenous nitroglycerin or milrinone (a phosphodiesterase inhibitor) infusion is commenced before the release of the aortic cross-clamp to enhance and maintain ITA and RA dilatation, protect against spasm, maximally dilate the coronary vascular bed for optimum graft runoff, and reduce the preload and, to a lesser degree, the afterload of the heart. Additionally, milrinone has an inotropic action. The following dosages are used: nitroglycerin, 0.5 to 2.5 µg/kg/min; milrinone, 0.1 to 0.2 µg/kg/min. The infusions are maintained for 24 hours, then switched to nitroglycerin topical paste, 25-mg slow-release patch for 24 hours, and additionally the calcium channel blocker felodipine, 2.5 to 5 mg orally daily.

We do not use calcium antagonist infusions (diltiazem) because these are not available in Australia. Additionally, there is some evidence that calcium channel blockers may be only partly effective,[25] with variable responses, (nifedipine is significantly more effective than diltiazem and verapamil),[26] and that nitrates (nitroglycerin and isosorbide dinitrate) are more effective in prophylaxis of RA graft spasm.

POSTOPERATIVE MANAGEMENT

Postbypass systolic pressure is kept at more than 110 mm Hg, mean arterial pressure more than 80 mm Hg, and the cardiac index at greater than 2.5 L/min/m^2. Systemic vascular resistance is maintained between 800 and 1,000 U. Aspirin is commenced within the first 24 hours and continued indefinitely. Patients are ambulated early (within 24 hours). The median discharge time is 5 days after surgery.

UNCONVENTIONAL RA CONDUIT USE
THE LITA-RA PEDICLE "Y" ("T") GRAFT

Some surgeons[8] believe that because the RA is a third-generation vessel, then its physiologic and hemodynamic milieu is best reproduced by anastomosis to the LITA. This maintains the concept of a pedicled graft, which in the ITA situation, has been generally associated with a higher patency rate. However, insufficient angiographic data exist to clearly indicate whether a "Y" graft or a direct aortocoronary graft is superior in long-term patency.

The proximal "Y" graft anastomosis should be constructed after heparinization but before cannulation and cardiopulmonary bypass. We favor a 7- to 8-mm arteriotomy on the anterior (chest wall) aspect of the LITA, at the level of the third intercostal branch (just as the ITA pedicle will later enter the pericardium via a slit anterior to the phrenic nerve). The end-to-side anastomosis is constructed in a parallel fashion with a continuous 7-0 polypropylene suture with a small (6-mm) needle, and the suture is tied as the ITA pedicle is released. (The distal LITA and RA are occluded with a small vascular clip.) The use of 6-0 polypropylene tacking sutures help support the RA pedicle on the LITA pedicle at and below the anastomosis, to prevent kinking. The length of RA pedicle gained by this technique is impressive, and it will readily reach the distal PDA in a normal-sized heart. When the LITA/RA "Y" pedicle is placed within the pericardium, the RA will have a gentle curve running initially inferiorly, then laterally, then posterolaterally to the circumflex territory. Alternatively, the "Y" anastomosis can be constructed on the fascial side of the LITA.[13,27]

If the first anastomosis with the RA "Y" is to a high marginal or intermediate artery, then the proximal ITA to RA "Y" graft anastomosis is placed higher on the ITA to ensure a smooth lie to the intermediate or high first marginal.

BILATERAL RA GRAFTS

When use of bilateral ITA grafts is impossible (prior damage or use), inappropriate (obesity, insulin-dependent diabetes), or insufficient for the required revascularization, or when there are insufficient other conduits (stripped veins, prior vascular or coronary procedure), then the harvesting of both RAs provides an abundance of excellent conduit,[28] allowing use of the LITA for the anterior wall, one RA for the lateral (circumflex) wall, and the other for the inferior (right coronary) wall. The use of bilateral RAs in association with ITAs allowed 98% of anastomoses to be constructed with arterial conduits.[9]

INABILITY TO USE RA

Radial artery dominance, 2% in our experience but up to 5%,[27] precludes its use.

Calcification of the RA can be so severe that it is a rigid pipe. Calcification of this severity occurs with an incidence of 2% to 3% (Fig 8). More frequent is patchy plaquelike calcification with flecks or plates up to 3 mm in diameter, particularly affecting the

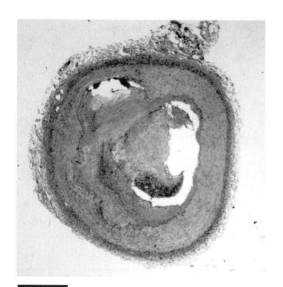

FIGURE 8.
A cross-section of a distal segment of radial artery showing a well-developed media, extensive calcification, and subtotal obliteration of the lumen.

distal portion and more extensive on the superficial side. If the calcification distally is extensive but confined, the proximal half or two thirds of the RA may be used, and the distal third is discarded. If the calcification is minor, then the RA can be used in such a way that the calcified areas are in the hood or dorsal surface of the RA conduit. If a judgment is made that the RA cannot be used (though partly mobilized), it is left intact in situ in the forearm.

Prior cannulation of the RA for arterial pressure monitoring may result in localized or extensive chronic dissection. Localized distal dissection of the RA is usually not recognized until the RA is being prepared and shaped for the distal anastomosis. The situation is usually managed by trimming off the distal 2 to 3 cm (removal of a localized dissection completely). More commonly, the RA appears perfectly normal after prior cannulation. In only one instance was the dissection so extensive as to preclude use of the graft.

We avoid RA use if there is known ipsilateral subclavian stenosis, prior trauma or surgery to the arm or forearm, or if the patient has advanced renal failure and may potentially require a forearm fistula for hemodialysis access.

CLINICAL DETAILS

The detailed data presented below are from our three interrelated institutions: The Royal Melbourne Hospital, the Austin and Repatriation Medical Centre (both teaching hospitals of the University

TABLE 2.

Patient Demographics for RA/CABG

Characteristics	Number
No. of patients	4,330
Age (yr)	64.3 ± 9.9
M/F	3,398:932 (78.5%:21.5%)
Angina class*	2.7 ± 1.1
Prior Q-wave myocardial infarction	1,766 (40.8%)
Unstable angina	1,223 (28.2%)
Left ventricular ejection fraction	
<0.50	1,134 (26.2%)
<0.30	144 (3.3%)
Diabetes	1,046 (24.2%)
Reoperation	289 (6.7%)

Note: Values are expressed in absolute numbers and percentages. Values are mean ± SD for age and angina class.

*Angina classification by Canadian Cardiovascular Society Classification.

Abbreviations: M, male; *F,* female.

of Melbourne, Australia), and Epworth Private Hospital in Melbourne. All data are prospectively collected onto a computer database and are subsequently available for analysis. The Society of Thoracic Surgery database definitions are used.

PATIENT DEMOGRAPHICS

From March 1995 to November 1998, 4,330 patients had isolated primary or redo CABG surgery in which at least one RA was used as part of the coronary reconstruction. Combined procedures (e.g., valve plus CABG) were excluded from this analysis.

A total of 5,381 RA graft conduits were used; 1,051 patients had both RAs used, and 3,279 patients had a single RA used.

The patient demographics are summarized in Table 2. The baseline characteristics are similar to prior reports with coronary surgery,[9,11,21] although others had used RAs in younger age groups (from 54.4 years to 60.2 years).[4,6-8] The incidence of diabetes mellitus had a trend to greater prevalence in patients in whom one and especially two RAs were used. Patients undergoing redo CABG are also more likely to receive RA grafts. Contraindications to RA use have been discussed above.

TRENDS IN RA USE

We commenced RA use in 1995, but with progressive familiarity with the harvest technique and conduit behavior, there was a rapid

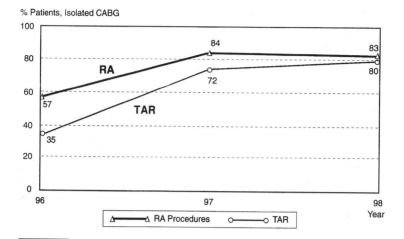

FIGURE 9.
Trends in radial artery (*RA*) use, and total arterial revascularization (*TAR*), 1996 to 1998. *Abbreviation: CABG,* coronary artery bypass graft.

escalation in RA use during 1996, and now the RA is at least one of the conduits in more than 80% of patients having CABG. The immediate effects on our practice have been to increase the rate of TAR to 80% by 1998 (Fig 9).

GRAFT USE

The LITA was used in 4,190 patients (96.7%). The RITA was used in 935 patients (21.6%), predominantly as a bilateral ITA procedure.

TABLE 3.
Details of Graft Use for Isolated CABG in 4,330 Patients (1995-1998)

Conduit	No. of Patients	%	No. of Distal Anastomoses	%
Radial	4,330	100	6,454	45.4
LITA	4,190	96.7	4,190	33.2
Sequential LITA	—	—	525	—
RITA (BITA)	935	21.6	935	6.7
Sequential RITA	—	—	16	—
Vein	1,515	34.9	2,082	14.7
TOTAL	4,330		14,202	

Abbreviation: BITA, bilateral internal thoracic artery.

TABLE 4.
Distribution of RAs: First RA (4,330 Patients)

Distal Vessel	Number of Patients	%	Anastomoses
LAD	91	2.1	91
DIAG	243	5.6	243
INT	36	0.8	36
Cx Marg	1,982	45.8	1,982
Sequential	753	17.4	1,657
RCA	148	3.4	148
PDA	935	21.6	935
LVBr	142	3.3	142
TOTAL	4,330	100	5,234

Abbreviations: DIAG, diagonal; INT, intermediate; Cx MARG, circumflex marginal; LVBr, left ventricular branch of the RCA.

Vein grafts were used in 1,515 patients (34.9%) accounting for 2,082 distal anastomoses. Hence, in this cohort, 75.1% of patients received arterial grafts only. Patterns of graft use are detailed in Table 3.

A total of 14,202 distal anastomoses were constructed (3.28 distal anastomoses per patient). RAs were used to construct 45.4% of all distal anastomoses, and arterial grafts only were used to construct 85.3% of all distal anastomoses (Table 3).

The patterns of use of the RA are detailed in Table 4 for the use of the first RA, and in Table 5 for the use of the second RA. The majority of the radial grafts were placed to the circumflex margin-

TABLE 5.
Distribution of Second RA in 1,051 Patients

Distal Vessel	No. of Patients	%	Anastomoses
LAD	14	1.3	14
DIAG/INT	24	2.3	24
Marginals	183	17.5	183
Sequential	143	13.7	312
RCA	69	6.6	69
PDA	514	48.8	514
LVBr	104	9.8	104
TOTAL	1,051	100	1,220

Abbreviations: LAD, left anterior descending coronary artery; DIAG, diagonal; INT, intermediate; RCA, right coronary artery; PDA, posterior descending artery; LVBr, left ventricular branch of the RCA.

TABLE 6.

Intraoperative Details

Variable	Number
Distal anastomoses per patient	3.28 ± 0.96
Total No. anastomoses	14,202
Aortic clamp time (min) (single aortic clamp for all distal and proximal anastomoses)	69.3 ± 24.2
Cardiopulmonary bypass time (min)	92.6 ± 35.5

Note: Values expressed are mean ± SD.

al system, although almost 30% went to the distal right coronary system. In addition, 17.4% of grafts were used in a sequential fashion, predominantly to the circumflex marginal system.

When a second RA was used, more than 65% of the distal anastomoses constructed with the second RA were to the distal right coronary system. When sequential grafting was used, 2.2 distal anastomoses were constructed per conduit.

OPERATIVE DETAILS

The intraoperative details are documented in Table 6. All distal and proximal anastomoses were performed during a single period of aortic cross-clamping. This technique was preferred to facilitate construction of the proximal anastomoses, and lessen the potential for trauma to the aorta and for embolization of particulate matter from the ascending aorta by minimizing aortic manipulation.

The ascending aorta was the most common site for the proximal RA anastomosis. Of 5,381 proximal anastomoses performed, the proximal RA anastomsis was constructed to the ascending aorta in 4,866 instances (90.4%), and to the LITA as a "Y" graft on 464 occasions (8.6%). An end-to-side anastomosis (Y) was constructed between two portions of RA (and rarely a vein) on 51 occasions (1.0%).

RESULTS

OPERATIVE MORTALITY

Forty-one patients died perioperatively or within the first 30 days of surgery. The perioperative and 30-day mortality was 0.9%, and did not differ between those having one or two RAs, or with our prior coronary experience.[9,11,21]

Acar et al.,[4] Brodman et al.,[16] Calafiore et al.,[8] Fremes et al.,[7] Da Costa et al.,[29] and Barner[30] report similar rates of perioperative mortality, ranging from 0% to 4.8%.

PERIOPERATIVE MORBIDITY

Sixty-nine patients (1.6%) had a stroke, defined as any neurologic abnormality producing motor, speech, or sensory deficits. Sixty-one patients (1.4%) had a sternal wound infection that required either intravenous antibiotics or reoperation to débride and rewire the sternum. Three patients required a muscle flap transfer. Twenty-five patients (0.6%) required reoperation for postoperative hemorrhage. There was only one reoperation because of bleeding from an RA branch. The low reoperation rate for hemorrhage has been an additional bonus from the use of the RA because the branches generally are small, are well-managed during the harvest process by small vascular clips, or diathermy, and are never the site of major or catastrophic bleeding. The bleeding rates are similar to those reported by Calafiore et al.[8] and lower than those reported by others.[25,29,30] In general, the rates of reoperation for bleeding when the RAs are used (0.4% to 2.4%) are generally lower than those reported for routine CABG surgery (4% to 5%).

PERIOPERATIVE MYOCARDIAL ISCHEMIA–INFARCTION, HYPOPERFUSION SYNDROME

Twenty-three patients (0.6%) had perioperative myocardial infarctions indicated by new Q waves or a creatinine kinase–MB (CKMB) level twice the upper limit of normal (normal value in our laboratory is 0-25 IU/L). The mean CKMB level 18 to 24 hours postoperatively was 15.4 ± 9.3 IU/L.

A hypoperfusion syndrome was rarely seen, with attention to pharmacologic dilatation of the ITAs and RAs during harvesting and preparation. Additionally, good myocardial protection is another important factor in minimizing poor cardiac performance postoperatively. An intra-aortic balloon was used in 26 patients (0.6%), predominantly when the patient was in a poor hemodynamic state preoperatively, had uncontrolled ischemic pain and ischemic electrocardiographic changes, or had a reoperation. In the literature, the average incidence of low cardiac output is reported to be 2.5%. The etiology of low cardiac output postoperatively, even in the setting of predominantly arterial (including RA) grafts, is multifactorial and is related to the preoperative state of the myocardium, myocardial protection, technical issues, native coronary spasm, and graft spasm. If arterial graft spasm is recognized, it should be managed by an additional graft (vein) to the same vessel or territory.[8] We believe there should be aggressive prophylactic management by atraumatic conduit handling, papaverine dilatation, liberal use of nitroglycerin or other vasodilators, and avoidance of postoperative hypotension. We do

TABLE 7.
Donor Forearm and Hand Complications in 4,330 Patients

Complications	Number
Hematoma (drainage)	9
Infection (drainage)	1
Infection (antibiotics)	12
Ischemia	2
TOTAL	24 (0.6%)

not use topical "ice slush" because this cold stimulus may be another causative factor for arterial graft spasm.

DONOR FOREARM AND HAND COMPLICATIONS
The incidence of donor forearm and hand complications is extremely low. There were only two instances (0.05%) of hand or finger ischemia (detailed above). The overall incidence of complications was less than 1% (Table 7). The forearm tissues healed well and rapidly, and there was excellent healing in the diabetic patients, who comprised 25% of the cohort. The incidence of reported forearm complications varies from 0% to 9%,[4,5,7,16,25,29] and these included nerve paresthesias. The avoidance of leg incisions avoided infection in that area (a significant problem in diabetic patients) and allowed rapid early ambulation.

DONOR FOREARM AND HAND FUNCTION
A total of 381 consecutive RA/CABG patients had a detailed functional assessment 3 months after surgery. Eighty-six patients (23%) had subjective numbness, 8 (2%) had an objective sensory deficit (monofilament sensation), 8 (2%) had weakness in the donor arm and below-average strength on objective assessment (although the donor arm was nondominant), and 67 (18%) had scar discomfort caused by either hypersensitivity or tightness (scar discomfort was the main complaint by patients). However, only 13 patients (3.5%) reported any interference with their normal activities 3 months postoperatively.

At review 6 months postoperatively, only 2 patients (0.5%) reported any residual discomfort. Objective measurements of muscle and power in the forearm and hand were only 5% less in the operated (nondominant) than in the nonoperated hand. The subjective and objective sensory abnormalities were both more prevalent in the distribution of the lateral cutaneous nerves of the forearm than in the SRN.

TABLE 8.
Graft Patency: RA in CABG

	% RA Graft Patent		
Report	Early (<3 mo)	Intermediate (1-2 yr)	Late (5 yr)
Acar et al.[31]	98%	90%	95%
Calafiore et al.[8]	99%	94%	—
Manasse et al.[25]	100% (but some diffuse changes)	84%	—
Da Costa et al.[29]	97%	100%	—
Chen et al.[6]	96%	—	—
Tatoulis et al.[9]	—	90%	—

Abbreviations: RA, radial artery; *CABG,* coronary artery bypass graft.

FOLLOW-UP

Apart from Carpentier and colleagues' early series from 1971, follow-up of RA/CABG patients is short, and most reports have concentrated on early clinical results. Dietl et al.[5] reported no deaths and no reoperations during a mean follow-up of 13 months, Da Costa et al.[29] reported one late death in 79 patients followed up for a mean of 10 months. Our own follow-up is also short, with a maximum of 36 months. The actuarial survival at 1 year was 97% ± 0.9%. However, it is not possible to reach meaningful inferences or conclusions with regard to the role of the RA in patient survival, apart from that it is not detrimental.

RA GRAFT PATENCY

Early patency (<3 months) is uniformly reported to be between 94% and 100%, and patency at 12 months reportedly is between 84% and 100%. Acar et al.[31] reported that 19 of 20 grafts (95%) were patent when studied at a mean of 5 years. A summary of reported RA graft patency is presented in Table 8.

We have studied 126 RA grafts and found 156 of 173 distal anastomoses (90%) to be patent at a mean of 9 months postoperatively. These graft studies were from a combination of a planned prospective angiographic study, or because of possible symptoms (Figs 10 through 14).

The degree of stenosis in the coronary artery being grafted may play a very important role. When the native vessel stenosis was greater than 70%, the patency rate was 94.6%. By comparison, when the native vessel stenosis was less than 70%, the RA paten-

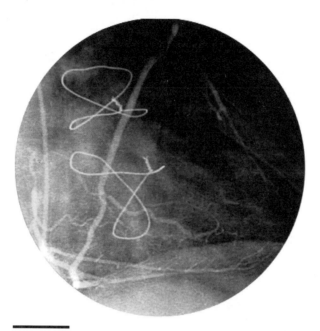

FIGURE 10.
RA graft anastomosed to the circumflex marginal and posterior descending coronary arteries.

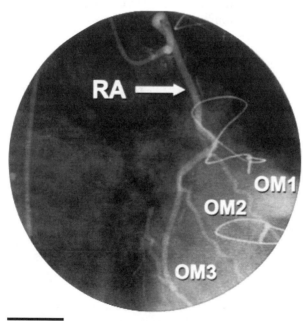

FIGURE 11.
Radial artery (*RA*) with sequential anastomoses to the first (*OM1*), second (*OM2*), and third (*OM3*) obtuse marginal arteries.

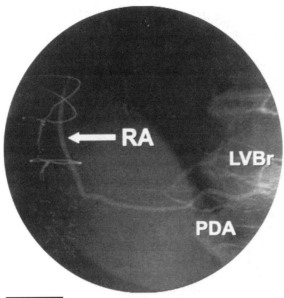

FIGURE 12.
Radial artery (*RA*) sequentially anastomosed side-to-side to the posterior descending artery (*PDA*), and end-to-side to the left ventricular branches (*LVBr*) of the right artery.

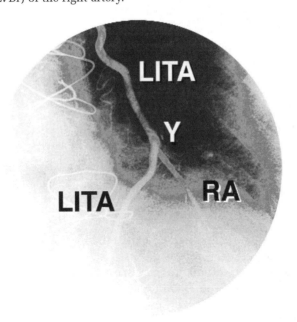

FIGURE 13.
A "Y" anastomosis between the left internal thoracic artery (*LITA*) and the radial artery (*RA*) to create a pedicled graft.

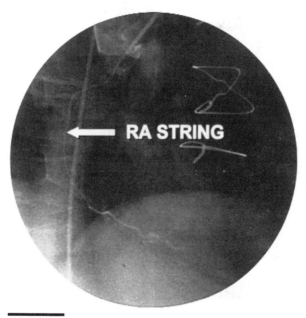

FIGURE 14.

A string sign in a radial artery (*RA*) anastomosed to the posterior descending coronary artery where the native right coronary artery was a large vessel with a 50% stenosis.

cy was 73% ($P < 0.002$). This reduction in patency and the development of a "string sign" in the face of less critical coronary anastomoses has been reported with RA grafts,[16] and also with free ITA grafts,[11] and may either represent the result of competitive flow or an autoregulatory mechanism.

Further meticulous long-term angiographic follow-up is essential to define the role of the RA. Although it would appear that once the RA is functioning normally in the coronary circulation free of technical and other problems, it has the potential to retain its patency in the long-term.

CONCLUSION

The RA is readily accessible and can be harvested in a majority of patients with coronary artery disease. It has excellent handling characteristics, abundant length and versatility, and allows uncompromised grafting distal to any stenosis or plaque. Conduit spasm can be overcome by meticulous surgical technique and preemptive pharmacologic vasodilation. The patency results are promising, and in our view, the RA will become the second graft of choice and allow widespread total arterial myocardial revascularization.

ACKNOWLEDGMENT

We would like to acknowledge the excellent assistance of Mrs. Jan Matthews and Miss Tonia Iacuone in the preparation of the manuscript, and Dr. Levent Efe for the original illustrations produced for this manuscript.

REFERENCES

1. Carpentier A, Guermontrez JL, Deloche A, et al: The aorta-to-coronary radial artery bypass graft: A technique avoiding pathological changes in grafts. *Ann Thorac Surg* 16:111-121, 1973.
2. Carpentier A: Discussion of Geha AS, Krone RJ, McCormack JR, et al: Selection of coronary bypass anatomic, physiological and angiographic considerations of vein and mammary artery grafts. *J Thorac Cardiovasc Surg* 70:404-431, 1975.
3. Curtis JJ, Stoney WS, Alford WC, et al: Intimal hyperplasia: A cause of radial artery aorto-coronary bypass graft failure. *Ann Thorac Surg* 20:628-635, 1975.
4. Acar C, Jebara VA, Portoghese M, et al: Revival of the radial artery for coronary artery bypass grafting. *Ann Thorac Surg* 54:652-660, 1992.
5. Dietl CA, Madigan NP, Menapace FJ, et al: Results of coronary artery bypass grafting using multiple arterial conduits. *J Cardiovasc Surg (Torino)* 34:513-516, 1993.
6. Chen AH, Nakao T, Brodman RS, et al: Eary post-operative angiographic assessment of radial artery grafts used for coronary artery bypass grafting. *J Thorac Cardiovasc Surg* 111:1208-1212, 1996.
7. Fremes SE, Christakis GT, Del Rizzo DF, et al: The technique of radial artery bypass grafting and early clinical results. *J Card Surg* 10:537-544, 1995.
8. Calafiore AM, Di Giammarco G, Teodori G, et al: Radial artery and inferior epigastric artery in composite grafts: Improved mid-term angiographic results. *Ann Thorac Surg* 60:517-524, 1995.
9. Tatoulis J, Buxton BF, Fuller JA: Bilateral radial artery grafts in coronary reconstruction: Techniques and early results in 261 patients. *Ann Thorac Surg* 66:714-720, 1998.
10. Loop FD, Lytle BW, Cosgrove DM, et al: Influence of the internal mammary artery graft on the 10 year survival and other cardiac events. *N Engl J Med* 204:1-6, 1986.
11. Tatoulis J, Buxton BF, Fuller JA: Results of 1454 free right internal thoracic artery-to-coronary artery grafts. *Ann Thorac Surg* 64:1263-1269, 1997.
12. Schmitt SE, Jones JW, Thornby JL, et al: Improved survival with multiple left sided bilateral internal thoracic artery grafts. *Ann Thorac Surg* 64:9-14, 1997.
13. Tector AJ, Amundsen S, Schmahl TM, et al: Total revascularization with "T" grafts. *Ann Thorac Surg* 57:33-39, 1994.
14. Kouchoukos NT, Wareing TH, Murphy SH, et al: Risks of bilateral internal mammary artery bypass grafting. *Ann Thorac Surg* 49:210-219, 1990.

15. Campeau L, Enjalbert M, Lestrance J, et al: Atherosclerosis and late closure of aorto-coronary saphenous vein graft: Sequential angiographic studies at 2 weeks, 1 year, 5-7 years and 10-12 years after surgery. *Circulation* 68:1S-7S, 1983.

16. Brodman RF, Frame R, Camacho M, et al: Routine use of unilateral and bilateral radial arteries for coronary bypass graft surgery. *J Am Coll Cardiol* 28:959-963, 1996.

17. Reyes AT, Frame R, Brodman RF: Techniques for harvesting the radial artery as a coronary bypass graft. *Ann Thorac Surg* 59:118-126, 1995.

18. McCormack LJ, Cauldwell EW, Anson BJ: Brachial and anti-brachial arterial patterns: A study of 750 extremities. *Surg Gynecol Obstet* 96: 43-54, 1953.

19. Little JM, Zylstra TI, West J, et al: Circulatory patterns in the normal hand. *Br J Surg* 60:652-655, 1973.

20. Kaufer E, Fasctor SM, Frame R, et al: Pathology of the radial and internal thoracic arteries used as coronary artery bypass grafts. *Ann Thorac Surg* 63:1118-1122, 1997.

21. Buxton BF, Fuller JA, Gaer J, et al: The radial artery as a bypass graft. *Curr Opin Cardiol* 11:591-598, 1996.

22. Chardigny C, Jebara VA, Acar C, et al: Vaso-reactivity of the radial artery: Comparison with the internal mammary and gastro-epiploic arteries, with implications for coronary artery surgery. *Circulation* 88: 115-127, 1993.

23. He GW, Yang CQ: Radial artery has higher receptor mediated contractility, but similar endothelial function compared with mammary artery. *Ann Thorac Surg* 63:1346-1352, 1997.

24. Liu JJ, Chen JR, Buxton BF: Unique response of human arteries to endothelium B receptor agonist and antagonist. *Clin Sci* 90:91-96, 1996.

25. Manasse CE, Sperti G, Suma H, et al: The use of the radial artery for myocardial revascularization. *Ann Thorac Surg* 52:1076-1083, 1996.

26. Cable DE, Caccitlo JA, Pearson PJ, et al: Approaches to prevention and treatment of radial artery graft vasospasms. *Circulation* 98:15S-22S, 1998.

27. Barner HB: Techniques of myocardial revascularization, in Edmunds LH (ed): *Cardiac Surgery in the Adult.* New York, McGraw-Hill, 1997, p 522.

28. Buxton BF, Fuller JA, Tatoulis J: Evolution of complete arterial grafting for coronary artery disease. *Tex Heart Inst J* 25:17-23, 1998.

29. Da Costa FDA, Da Costa IA, Poffo R, et al: Myocardial revascularization with the radial artery: A clinical and angiographic study. *Ann Thorac Surg* 62: 475-480, 1996.

30. Barner HB: Defining the role of the radial artery. *Semin Thorac Cardiovasc Surg* 8:3-9, 1996.

31. Acar C, Jebara V, Fabiani J, et al: Radial artery: Surgical techniques and clinical results, in Angelini G, Bryan A, Dion R (eds): *Arterial Conduits in Myocardial Revascularization.* London, Arnold, 1996, pp 141-146.

CHAPTER 6

Aortic Valve Repair for Management of Aortic Insufficiency

Tirone E. David, M.D.
Professor of Surgery, University of Toronto; Head, Division of
Cardiovascular Surgery, The Toronto Hospital, Toronto, Ontario, Canada

A ortic valve repair is not a commonly performed operation in the management of aortic insufficiency (AI). At The Toronto Hospital, from 1990 to 1998, 834 patients had surgery for native aortic valve insufficiency: 223 (27%) had aortic valve repair, and 611 (73%) had aortic valve replacement. To perform aortic valve repair for AI, the cardiac surgeon must have a thorough understanding of the functional anatomy of the aortic valve. Thus, the functional anatomy of the aortic valve, as well as the pathology and pathophysiology of AI, are reviewed first, followed by a discussion of aortic valve repair.

FUNCTIONAL ANATOMY OF AORTIC VALVE

The morphology and function of the aortic valve are intimately related to the aortic root, and they are best described as a single functional unit. The aortic root connects the left ventricle with the ascending aorta. The aortic root has four anatomical components: the aortoventricular junction or aortic annulus, the leaflets, the aortic sinuses or sinuses of Valsalva, and the sinotubular junction.

The aortic root is attached to ventricular muscle in approximately 45% of its circumference and to fibrous structures (mitral valve and membranous septum) in the remaining 55% (Fig 1). Histologic examination of the aortoventricular junction reveals that the aortic root has a fibrous continuity with the anterior leaflet of the mitral valve and membranous septum, and it is attached to the muscular interventricular septum through fibrous strands (Fig 2). Because the entire

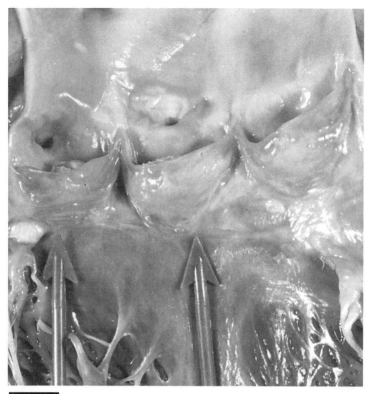

FIGURE 1.

A photograph of the left ventricular outflow tract and the aortic root. The aortic root is attached to ventricular muscle in approximately 45% of its circumference and to fibrous tissue in 55%. The *left arrow* points to the lateral fibrous trigone below the left coronary leaflet. The *right arrow* points to the junction of the membranous and muscular interventricular septum below the right coronary leaflet.

circumference of the aortic root contains connective tissue where it is attached to the left ventricle, it is reasonable to refer to the aortoventricular junction as aortic annulus.

The aortic leaflets are attached to the aortic root in a semilunar fashion. The segments of arterial wall of the aortic root delineated by the leaflets proximally and by the sinotubular junction distally are called aortic sinuses or sinuses of Valsalva. There are three aortic leaflets and sinuses: the left, the right, and the noncoronary. The left main coronary artery arises from the left aortic sinus and the right coronary artery arises from the right aortic sinus. The left main coronary artery orifice is closer to the aortic annulus than the right coronary artery orifice. The triangular space underneath two leaflets is part of the left ventricle. The highest point of this triangle where two

A　　　　　　**B**

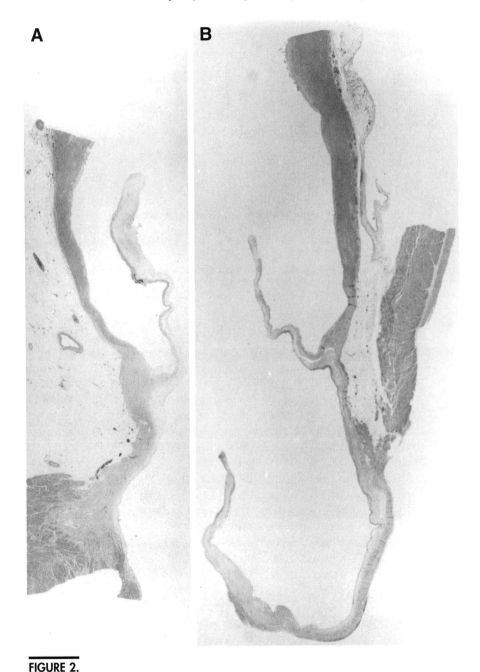

FIGURE 2.
A, a photomicrograph of the aortoventricular junction along the right coronary sinus and muscular ventricular septum. Connective tissue unites the aortic root to the ventricular septum. **B,** a photomicrograph of the aortoventricular junction along the noncoronary aortic sinus. There is a fibrous continuity between the aortic valve and mitral valve (the intervalvular fibrous body).

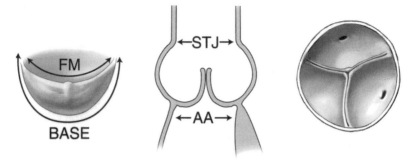

FIGURE 3.
Geometric relationships of the components of the aortic root. The length of the base of the aortic leaflet is approximately 1.5 times longer than the length of the free margin (*FM*). The diameter of the aortic annulus (*AA*) is approximately 15% to 20% larger than the diameter of the sinotubular junction (*STJ*). The FMs of the leaflets extend from commissure to commissure, and the commissures are immediately below the STJ. Therefore, the diameter of the STJ cannot exceed the length of the FM of the leaflets.

leaflets are attached is called the commissure and is located immediately below the sinotubular junction. The two triangular spaces underneath the commissures of the noncoronary leaflet are fibrous structures, whereas the triangular space underneath the commissure between the right and left leaflets is mostly a muscular structure (myocardium). These triangles can be seen in Figure 1. The sinotubular junction represents the end of the aortic root and is an important structure because the commissures of the leaflets are located immediately below it. Changes in the diameter of the sinotubular junction affect the motion and coaptation of the aortic leaflets.

The geometry of the aortic root and its anatomical components vary somewhat from person to person, but the geometric relationships among the various components are fairly constant in an individual. Thus, the sizes of the aortic leaflets determine the diameters of the aortic annulus and of the sinotubular junction, as well as the sizes of the sinuses of Valsalva. Each aortic leaflet has a crescentic shape, and the length of its base is approximately 1.5 times longer than the length of its free margin (Fig 3). The lengths of the free margins vary from leaflet to leaflet in an individual, but the noncoronary leaflet is often the largest of the three, followed by the right leaflet. The lengths of the free margins of the leaflets and the diameter of the aortic annulus are interrelated.[1] Because the free margin of a leaflet extends from one commissure to another, the diameter of the aortic annulus cannot exceed the average lengths of the free margins of the leaflets, as illustrated in Figure 3. The diameter of the aortic annulus is 15% to 20% larger than the diameter of the sinotubular junction.[1]

The anatomical relationships between the aortic root and surrounding structures are also important for cardiac surgeons. The right aortic sinus relates with the pulmonary root, right ventricular outflow tract, and body of the right ventricle. The subcommissural triangle between the right and noncoronary leaflets is in contact with the right atrium. The proximal part of the noncoronary aortic sinus relates with the dome of the left atrium and with the right atrium. The left aortic sinus relates mostly with the dome of the left atrium.

The aortic root is attached to contractile and fibrous components of the left ventricle. During systole, the interventricular septum shortens and moves inward, and the anterior leaflet of the mitral valve is pushed away from the center of the left ventricular outflow tract. Thus, during systole, the area of the aortic root that is attached to the anterior leaflet of the mitral valve is exposed to greater tension than the area attached to the muscular interventricular septum. These dynamic changes in the geometry of the aortic annulus play a role in function of the aortic valve. Although all three aortic leaflets open synchronously during systole, the noncoronary leaflet, and its annulus and commissures are exposed to greater stress (LaPlace's law). This may explain why the noncoronary aortic sinus and its annulus tend to dilate more than the other sinuses in patients with degenerative disease of the aorta.

The sinuses of Valsalva are important to maintain coronary artery blood flow throughout the cardiac cycle as well as to create eddies currents to close the aortic leaflets during diastole (Fig 4). The aortic root is very elastic in young patients and expands considerably dur-

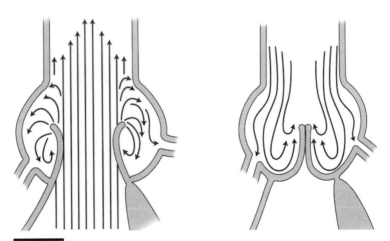

FIGURE 4.
Closure of the aortic valve is facilitated by eddies currents created by the aortic sinuses. The aortic sinuses are also important to guarantee coronary artery perfusion during systole.

ing systole and shortens during diastole. However, the number of elastic fibers in the aortic root (and elsewhere in the aorta) decreases with age, and the aortic root becomes less compliant in older patients; it expands minimally during systole in elderly patients.

PATHOLOGY OF AORTIC INSUFFICIENCY

From January 1990 to August 1998, 834 patients with native aortic valve insufficiency underwent aortic valve surgery at The Toronto Hospital. Table 1 shows the incidence of the various diseases that caused AI in this group of patients.

Bicuspid aortic valve disease is common and probably occurs in 1% to 2% of the population. A bicuspid aortic valve usually functions satisfactorily and does not cause hemodynamic problems until late in life when it becomes calcified and stenotic. It can also cause AI in younger patients, in which case it is frequently associated with dilatation of the aortic annulus and root.[2] Most patients with bicuspid aortic valves have three aortic sinuses. The two leaflets are of different size, and the larger one usually has a raphe instead of a commissure. This raphe extends from the midportion of the leaflet to the aortic annulus, and its insertion in the aortic root is often at a lower level than the other two commissures. Bicuspid aortic valve with two aortic sinuses and no raphe is uncommon. The left coronary artery is dominant in most patients with bicuspid aortic valve disease.

Unicusp aortic valve is less common than bicuspid aortic valve and seldom causes AI. It is characterized by the presence of only one commissure and often causes aortic stenosis.

Both unicuspid and bicuspid aortic valves are congenital anomalies of the aortic root that are often associated with premature degenerative changes of the media of the wall of the aortic root and ascending aorta. These patients are at risk of developing chronic degenerative aneurysm of the ascending aorta as well as type A aortic dissection.[3]

Quadricusp aortic valve may also cause AI. Three cusps are usually of similar size and one is hypoplastic.

Subaortic membraneous ventricular septal defect can cause AI because of distortion of the aortic annulus and leaflet prolapse. Initially the leaflet prolapse is caused by distortion of the annulus alone, but with time its free margin may become elongated and aggravate the degree of prolapse, with worsening of AI.

Dilatation of the sinotubular junction is a common cause of AI. The aortic valve can be bicuspid or tricuspid in these patients.[4,5] In our experience, older patients with ascending aortic aneurysms and AI frequently have an aortic annulus of normal diameter, a tricuspid aortic valve with normal or minimally diseased leaflets, and the AI is largely caused by dilatation of the sinotubular junc-

TABLE 1.
Pathology of AI in 834 Patients

Annuloaortic ectasia	257	(31%)
Annuloaortic ectasia + bicuspid aortic valve	50	(6%)
Annuloaortic ectasia + other congenital aortic valve disease	1	
Annuloaortic ectasia + dissection	6	
Annuloaortic ectasia + rheumatic	3	
Dilated sinotubular junction	49	(6%)
Bicuspid aortic valve	125	(15%)
Bicuspid aortic valve + dissection	8	
Bicuspid aortic valve + rheumatic	13	
Other congenital (quadricuspid, other)	18	(2%)
Other congenital + dissection	1	
Rheumatic	163	(19%)
Dissection (acute or chronic)	69	(8%)
Other tricuspid valve disease		
Infective endocarditis	23	(3%)
Nonspecific inflammatory	14	(2%)
Ventricular septal defect + prolapse	9	(1%)
Isolated prolapse	3	
Unknown	22	(3%)

tion. In younger patients, the aneurysms tend to be more proximal and involve the sinuses of Valsalva, the aortic annulus (annuloaortic ectasia), and the sinotubular junction. This type of pathology is encountered in patients with the Marfan syndrome or its forma frusta. Dilatation of the aortic root is the most common cause of AI in our series (Table 1) as well as in others.[4]

Aortic dissections involving the ascending aorta can cause AI because of preexisting dilatation of the aortic root and/or by detachment of one or more commissures with consequent prolapse of the leaflets.

Ankylosing spondylitis, Reiter's syndrome, osteogenesis imperfecta, rheumatoid arthritis, systemic lupus erythematosus, and idiopathic giant cell aortitis are connective tissue disorders that can be associated with AI. The anorexigenic drugs phenteramine and fenfluramine can also cause AI.

PATHOPHYSIOLOGY OF AORTIC INSUFFICIENCY

AI is caused by anatomical abnormalities of one or more components of the aortic root. Dilatation of the sinotubular junction causes outward displacement of the commissures of the aortic leaflets and prevents central coaptation, resulting in AI (Fig 5). This is the mecha-

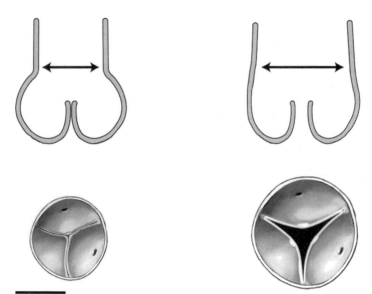

FIGURE 5.
Dilation of the sinotubular junction causes outward displacement of the commissures of the aortic valve and prevents the leaflets from coapting, with resulting central AI.

nism of AI in patients with ascending aortic aneurysms, mega-aorta syndrome, and in those with long-standing hypertension and a mildly dilated and elongated ascending aorta. Depending on the duration of AI, rapidity of dilation, and leaflet strength, the leaflets may remain grossly normal, or the free margin of one or more leaflets may become elongated or may develop fenestrations in the commissural areas. These changes in the leaflets are probably secondary to increased mechanical stress resulting from lack of coaptation.

Dilatation of the sinuses of Valsalva does not cause AI if the aortic annulus and the sinotubular junction remain normal. That is why patients with a ruptured sinus of Valsalva aneurysm may not have AI.

Patients with Marfan syndrome and those with the forma frusta of Marfan syndrome initially have dilatation of the aortic sinuses only, with no change in the diameters of the sinotubular junction and aortic annulus. Most of these patients have no AI until the diameter of the sinuses of Valsalva reaches 45 to 50 mm, at which point the sinotubular junction dilates, the aortic leaflets can no longer coapt, and central AI ensues. The aortic annulus may also dilate and contributes to the pathophysiology of AI in these patients. The fibrous components of the left ventricular outflow tract become enlarged, and the normal relationship between muscular (45% of the circumference) and fibrous components (55% of the circumference) is altered in favor of the fibrous component.

Bicuspid aortic valves cause AI because of leaflet prolapse. The free margin of the larger of the two leaflets, usually the one that contains the raphe, becomes elongated and prolapses. These patients often have dilatation of the aortic root, with increased diameters of the aortic annulus and sinotubular junction.

Type A aortic dissection causes AI because of detachment of one or both commissures of the noncoronary leaflet of the aortic valve, with resulting prolapse. In addition, most of these patients have preexisting dilatation of the aortic root, which contributes to the pathophysiology of AI.

Rheumatic valvulitis of the aortic valve can cause commissural fusion, thickening, scarring, and contraction of the leaflets, which are inadequate to seal the aortic valve orifice. Some degree of aortic stenosis is almost always present in these cases. Rheumatic AI is commonly associated with rheumatic mitral valve disease.

Although infective endocarditis of the aortic valve is far more common in patients with preexisting aortic valve disease, a normally functioning tricuspid aortic valve can become infected, resulting in leaflet destruction and AI.

Subaortic membranous ventricular septal defect causes AI because of down and outward displacement of the aortic annulus along the right leaflet that, with time, may become elongated and increase the degree of leaflet prolapse.

PREOPERATIVE SELECTION OF PATIENTS FOR AORTIC VALVE REPAIR

A more aggressive approach in the treatment of AI and aortic root aneurysm is probably justifiable if the native aortic valve can be saved. Therefore, it is important to determine the feasibility of aortic valve repair in these patients.

Transesophageal echocardiography is the best tool to study the aortic root and the mechanism of AI. The echocardiographer must understand the functional anatomy of the aortic root and the principles of aortic valve repair to obtain the information needed to determine the probability of successfully repairing the aortic valve. Each component of the aortic root must be examined, particularly the leaflets. Calcification of the aortic annulus and subannular regions indicates a more advanced degenerative process that often preclu aortic valve repair. Subaortic membranous ventricular septal ect deforms the aortic annulus of the right aortic leaflet, and in adult patient, the leaflet may be calcified. The number of l ets, their thickness, the appearance of their free margins, and t' excursion of each leaflet during the cardiac cycle must be caref examined. The coaptation areas of the leaflets should als interrogated by Doppler echocardiography in multiple view mation regarding the morphology of the aortic sinuses, s. ular junction, and

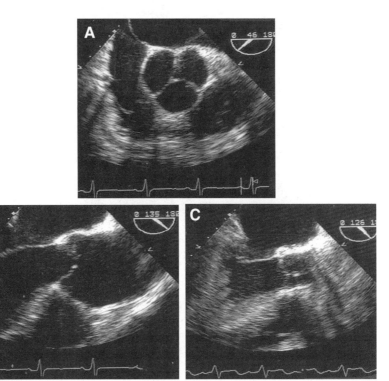

FIGURE 6.
Echocardiographic photographs of the aortic root of a patient with mega-aorta syndrome, aortic root aneurysm, and severe AI **(A)**. The leaflets do not coapt centrally **(B)**. Remodeling of the sinotubular junction of the aortic root with a tubular Dacron graft restored valve competence **(C)**.

ascending aorta is also important. The diameters of the aortic annulus, aortic sinuses, sinotubular junction, and the heights of the leaflets should be measured. The lengths of the free margins of the leaflets should be estimated if possible.

Dilatation of the sinotubular junction is easily diagnosed by echocardiography. If the aortic sinuses, leaflets, and annulus appear to be normal by echocardiography, and the AI is central (Fig 6, A and B), reconstruction of the aortic root with preservation of the aortic valve will restore normal valve function (Fig 6, C).[6] Patients with dilated sinotubular junction are frequently in their sixth and seventh decades of life, often have history of hypertension, and have degenerative aneurysm of the ascending aorta or mega-aorta syndrome.

Dilatation of the entire aortic root with AI as found in patients with the Marfan syndrome or its forma frusta is also a correctable lesion, providing the leaflets are normal or near normal (Fig 7). In patients with large aortic root aneurysms (diameter of the aortic

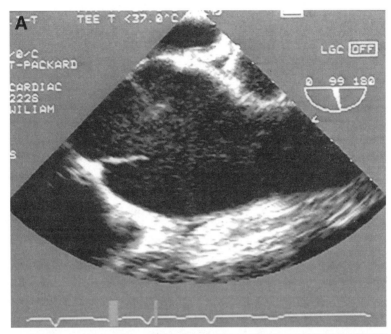

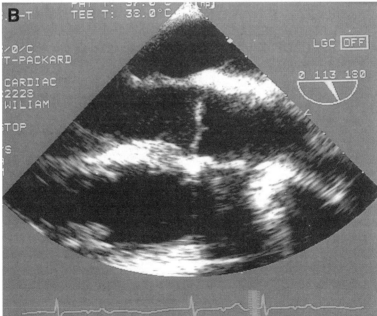

FIGURE 7.
Echocardiographic photographs of the aortic root of a patient with the Marfan syndrome, aortic root aneurysm, and severe AI with normal leaflets **(A)**. Remodeling of the aortic root with replacement of all three aortic sinuses restored valve competence **(B)**.

sinuses greater than 60 mm), the leaflets may be overstretched, thinned, and have large stress fenestrations in the commissural areas. Although fenestrations are not detected by echocardiography, a regurgitant jet in a commissural area in these patients usually indicates a large fenestration. The leaflets are often normal or minimally stretched in patients with aortic root aneurysms of 55 mm or less in diameter. However, even in patients with larger aneurysms, if the AI is only central and no leaflet prolapses, a valve-sparing operation is feasible.

AI caused by prolapse of a single leaflet in patients with a normal aortic root is uncommon but easily repairable. Prolapse of one leaflet in patients with bicuspid aortic valve is more common and also amenable to repair, as long as the leaflets are thin, mobile, and free from calcification.

Echocardiography has not been useful in predicting the feasibility of repair of rheumatic aortic valves, but it is useful in ruling it out.

OPERATIVE TECHNIQUE

Aortic valve repair must be performed with intraoperative transesophageal Doppler echocardiography. An attempt should be made to establish the mechanism of AI by Doppler echocardiography, and all diameters of the aortic root are obtained again before placing the patient on cardiopulmonary bypass. With the exception of patients with acute type A aortic dissection in whom cardiopulmonary bypass is established by cannulating a femoral artery and the right atrium, we always insert the arterial cannula in the ascending aorta or transverse aortic arch and the venous cannula in the right atrium in patients with AI. The aorta is opened transversely 1 to 2 cm above the sinotubular junction. The myocardium is protected by continuous antegrade blood cardioplegia through Polystan coronary artery cannulas (Polystan A/S Vaerlose, Denmark) placed directly into the main coronary artery orifices. A left ventricular vent is inserted through the right superior pulmonary vein and mitral valve to obtain a dry operative field.

Intraoperatively, the mechanism of AI is established by careful surgical inspection of each component of the aortic root. Because the feasibility of aortic valve repair is highly dependent on the quality and morphology of the aortic leaflets, they are inspected first. If the aortic valve is tricuspid, the leaflets are thin and pliable, and inspection of each leaflet reveals that they have their typical crescentic shape, aortic valve repair is likely feasible. Next, the three commissures should be gently suspended with forceps or sutures at approximately the same level and equidistantly to allow the leaflets to coapt, to determine whether the free margin of any of the three leaflets is elongated and prolapsing. If the leaflets coapt normally, the AI must be caused by dilatation of the sinotubular junction. If one leaflet coapts at a lower level than the other two, its free margin is elongated and it should be shortened before proceeding with the next step of the valve repair. The same patient may have AI caused by leaflet prolapse and dilatation of the sinotubular junction and/or of the aortic annulus.

REPAIR OF LEAFLET PROLAPSE

Prolapse of a single leaflet in patients with tricuspid aortic valve is corrected by either a triangular resection or plication of the central portion of the leaflet to shorten its free margin. The degree of shortening is based on the length of the free margins of the other two leaflets to allow them to coapt at the same level. If the leaflet is myxomatous and thickened, we perform a triangular resection and approximate the margins with interrupted horizontal mattress sutures of 5-0 polypropylene buttressed on two small strips of autologous pericardium. If the leaflet is thin and overstretched, we perform a triangular plication with the same type of suture. Figure 8 illustrates this operative technique.

Minor elongation of the free margin of a leaflet can also be corrected with a double layer of 6-0 Gore-Tex suture (W.L. Gore & Associates, Langstaff, Ariz) passed along the free margin from commissure to commissure (Fig 9). This technique allows for a fine band of fibrous tissue to grow along the suture and surrounding leaflet tissue, reinforcing its free margin. We often use this technique in patients with AI caused by dilatation of the aortic root in whom one leaflet is slightly more elongated than the other two, and it is thin and overstretched. We also use it to reinforce the free margins when large fenestrations are found.

If the aortic root is normal, repair of the leaflet prolapse is all that is required to correct the AI. If the aortic root is dilated, remodeling of the aortic root is also necessary.

REPAIR OF INCOMPETENT BICUSPID AORTIC VALVE

Incompetent bicuspid aortic valves can be satisfactorily repaired when both leaflets are pliable without calcification, the AI is caused by prolapse of only one leaflet, and the aortic root is only mildly dilated. The leaflet that contains the raphe is the larger of the two and often the one that prolapses. The raphe should be resected, and a triangular plication of the central portion of the free margin is performed to shorten its length (Fig 10). If the aortic annulus is mildly dilated, plication of the triangular space underneath the commissure reduces the diameter of the aortic annulus and increases the coaptation area of the two leaflets (Fig 11).

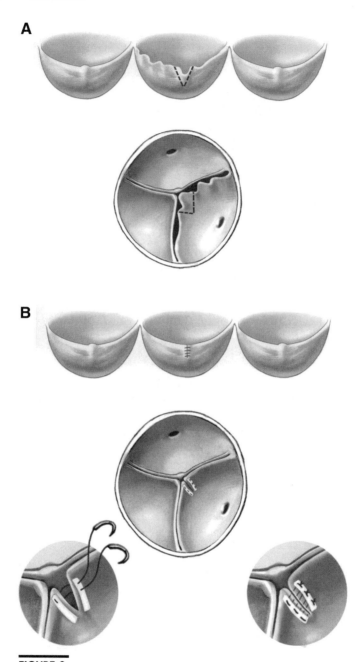

FIGURE 8.
AI caused by leaflet prolapse. The free margin of one leaflet is longer than the other two **(A)**. Triangular resection of the central portion of the prolapsing leaflet and reapproximation of the resected margins with horizontal mattressed sutures corrects the prolapse **(B)**. Alternatively, plication of a triangular segment of the central portion can also be performed.

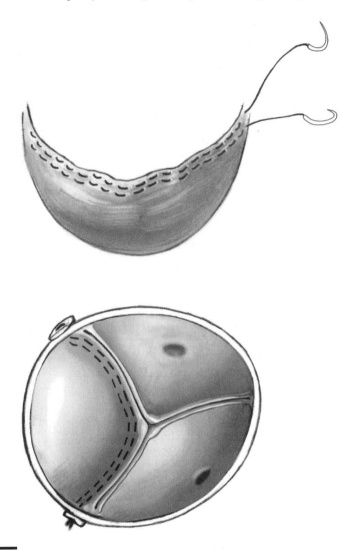

FIGURE 9.
The free margin of a leaflet can be reinforced and mild prolapse can be corrected with a double layer of 6-0 Gore-Tex suture from commissure to commissure.

REMODELING OF AORTIC ROOT FOR DILATATION OF SINOTUBULAR JUNCTION

Dilatation of the sinotubular junction displaces the commissures outward and prevents the leaflets from coapting during diastole (Fig 5). Dilatation is often more severe along the area of the non-coronary aortic sinus. Patients with dilated sinotubular junctions and AI frequently have aneurysms of the ascending aorta. AI can

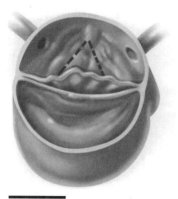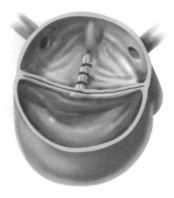

FIGURE 10.
Repair of incompetent bicuspid aortic valve: the raphe is resected and the prolapsing leaflet is shortened by triangular resection or plication of the central portion of the free margin.

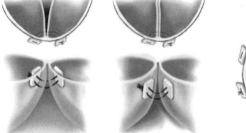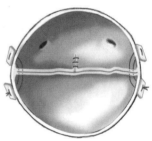

FIGURE 11.
Repair of bicuspid aortic valve: plication of the subcommissural triangles increases the coaptation areas of the two leaflets and reduces the diameter of the aortic annulus.

be corrected by reducing the sinotubular junction to its normal diameter. This is accomplished by replacing the ascending aorta with a tubular Dacron graft with a diameter that is slightly smaller than the average length of the free margins of the three leaflets, and suturing the graft right at the sinotubular junction (Fig 12). The three commissures of the aortic valve should be equidistantly placed in the Dacron graft if all three leaflets have similar sizes. If one leaflet is larger than the others, the space between its commissures should be proportionally larger. The Dacron graft should lie against the intima of the aortic root along the suture line at the level of the sinotubular junction and secured to it with a simple continuous 4-0 polypropylene suture in a fine cardiovascular nee-

Patients With a Normal Aortic Annulus

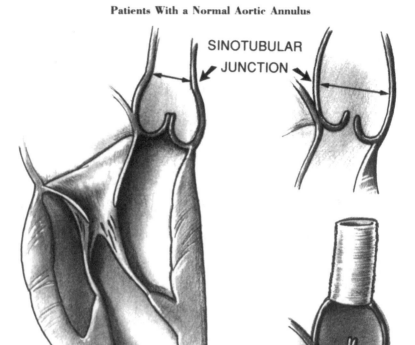

SINOTUBULAR
JUNCTION

FIGURE 12.
Remodeling of the aortic root by correcting the dilated sinotubular junction. This is accomplished by replacing the ascending aorta with a tubular Dacron graft with a diameter that is 5% to 10% smaller than the average lengths of the free margins of the leaflets. (Reproduced from David TE, Feindel CM, Bos J: Repair of the aortic valve in patients with aortic insufficiency and aortic root aneurysm. *J Thorac Cardiovasc Surg* 109:345-352, 1995.)

dle. This suture should be interrupted at each commissure. We have not used Teflon felt to buttress this suture line. If the estimated diameter of the sinotubular junction is less than 24 mm, it is preferable to use a Dacron graft with a larger diameter (e.g., 26 or 28 mm) and reduce one of its ends to the desirable diameter before suturing it to the sinotubular junction of the aortic root, to avoid a mismatch between the size of the graft and the size of the patient. Small-diameter grafts in the ascending aorta can be obstructive and cause an increase in left ventricular afterload.

In addition to a dilated sinotubular junction, one or more sinuses of Valsalva may also be aneurysmal. The noncoronary sinus of Valsalva is the most commonly affected in patients with ascending aortic aneurysms and dilated sinotubular junctions. If the other two sinuses are fairly normal, only the dilated aortic sinus needs replacement. Selecting a graft of appropriate diameter (5% to 10% smaller than the average lengths of the free margins of the three aortic leaflets) and tailoring one of its ends to replace the noncoronary aortic sinus does this. If all three leaflets have similar sizes, one of the ends of the graft is divided in three equal thirds and a sinus is tailored in one of the ends of the Dacron graft (Fig 13). The height of the Dacron sinus is approximately equal to the diameter of the graft. The graft is sutured to the sinotubular junction of the aortic root along the left and right aortic sinuses and to the remnants of the noncoronary sinus and part of the aortic annu-

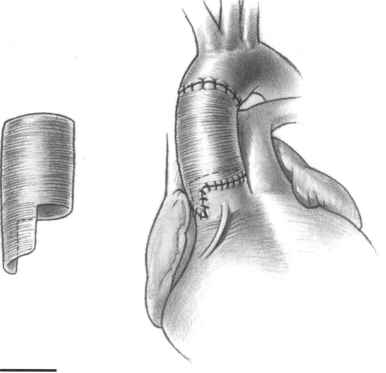

FIGURE 13.
Remodeling of the aortic root by correcting the dilated sinotubular junction and replacing the noncoronary aortic sinus. (Reproduced from David TE, Feindel CM, Bos J: Repair of the aortic valve in patients with aortic insufficiency and aortic root aneurysm. *J Thorac Cardiovasc Surg* 109:345-352, 1995.

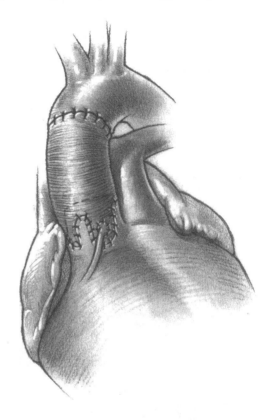

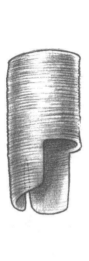

FIGURE 14.
Remodeling of the aortic root by correcting the dilated sinotubular junction and replacing the noncoronary and the right aortic sinuses. (Reproduced from David TE, Feindel CM, Bos J: Repair of the aortic valve in patients with aortic insufficiency and aortic root aneurysm. *J Thorac Cardiovasc Surg* 109:345-352, 1995.)

lus. The graft should lie against the intima of the aortic root along the suture line.

The right aortic sinus is the second most commonly involved and may need replacement during remodeling of the aortic root. In this case, the right coronary artery has to be reimplanted (Fig 14).

In most patients with aortic root aneurysm, all three aortic sinuses are dilated and need replacement. This is performed by excising all three aortic sinuses and replacing them with a properly tailored Dacron graft (Figs 15, 16, and 17).

REMODELING OF AORTIC ROOT FOR DILATATION OF AORTIC ANNULUS

In patients with AI, dilatation of the aortic annulus or annuloaortic ectasia is seldom seen in isolation and is often associated with

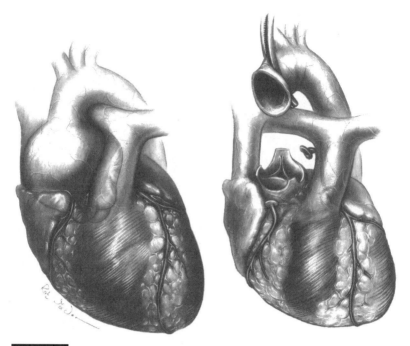

FIGURE 15.
Remodeling of the aortic root by replacing all three aortic sinuses. All three aortic sinuses are excised. (Reproduced from David TE: Remodeling of the aortic root and preservation of the native aortic valve. *Op Tech Cardiac Thorac Surg* 1:44-56, 1996.)

dilatation of the sinotubular junction and aortic root aneurysm. These patients may or may not have Marfan syndrome. The aortic leaflets are often normal or near normal in these patients when the aortic root is not excessively large. We believe that remodeling of the aortic root must include correction of the dilated aortic annulus. The diameter of the aortic annulus should not exceed the average length of the free margins of the aortic leaflets. Dilatation of the aortic annulus occurs along its fibrous component. Correction of dilatation of the aortic annulus can be accomplished by an aortic annuloplasty. This is performed by passing multiple horizontal mattress sutures of 4-0 or 3-0 polyester from the inside to the outside of the fibrous component of the left ventricular outflow tract immediately below the lowest level of the insertion of the leaflets through a single horizontal plane (Fig 18). These sutures are then passed through a strip of Dacron fabric to reduce the diameter of the aortic annulus, especially underneath the commissures of the noncoronary leaflet. The length of the strip of Dacron fabric is based on the desired diameter of the aortic annulus, calculated by

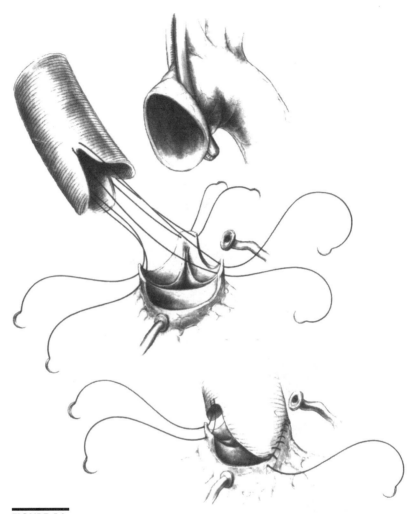

FIGURE 16.
Remodeling of the aortic root by replacing all three aortic sinuses. A properly tailored tubular Dacron graft is used to resuspend the three aortic commissures and replace the aortic sinuses. (Reproduced from David TE: Remodeling of the aortic root and preservation of the native aortic valve. *Op Tech Cardiac Thorac Surg* 1:44-56, 1996.)

measuring the lengths of the free margins of the aortic leaflets. The aortic sinuses and ascending aorta are replaced as described above (Figs 16, 17, and 19).

REIMPLANTATION OF AORTIC VALVE
Another method of correcting annuloaortic ectasia and AI is reimplantation of the aortic valve. The aortic root is dissected circum-

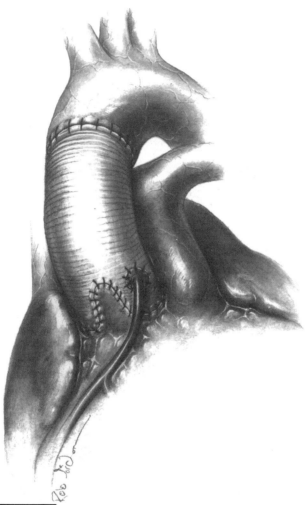

FIGURE 17.
Remodeling of the aortic root with replacement of all three aortic sinuses.
The coronary arteries are reimplanted in their respective aortic sinuses.
(Reproduced from David TE: Remodeling of the aortic root and preserva-
tion of the native aortic valve. *Op Tech Cardiac Thorac Surg* 1:44-56,
1996.)

ferentially and all three dilated aortic sinuses are excised, leaving
a small button of arterial wall around the coronary artery orifices
and some arterial wall attached to the aortic annulus. Multiple
sutures of 4-0 or 3-0 polyester are passed from the inside to the
outside of the left ventricular outflow tract. This suture line is in a
single horizontal plane along the fibrous component of the left
ventricular outflow tract, and it follows the scalloped shape of the

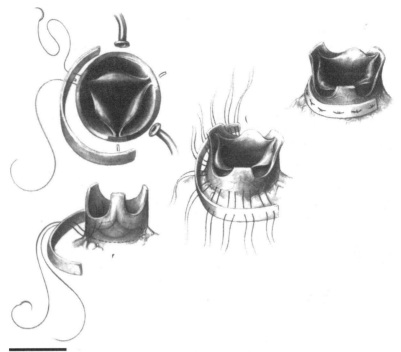

FIGURE 18.
Aortic annuloplasty to correct annuloaortic ectasia in patients with dilated aortic annulus and aortic root aneurysm. Multiple horizontal mattress sutures are passed through the fibrous components of the left ventricular outflow tract, through a single horizontal plane immediately below the lowest level of the leaflets. (Reproduced from David TE: Remodeling of the aortic root and preservation of the native aortic valve. *Op Tech Cardiac Thorac Surg* 1:44-56, 1996.)

aortic annulus in its muscular component (Fig 20). A tubular Dacron graft with a diameter equal to the average length of the free margins of the three aortic leaflets is selected. Three equidistant marks are made in one of its ends, and the scalloped shape of the suture line in the left ventricular outflow tract is tailored in the Dacron graft (Fig 20). These sutures are then passed from the inside to the outside of the Dacron graft. They must be equidistantly distributed, and reduction in the diameter of the aortic annulus is accomplished underneath the commissures of the non-coronary leaflet—that is, the sutures are spaced closer together in the graft than they are spaced in the left ventricular outflow tract. The valve is placed inside the graft, and all sutures are tied on the outside. Next, the three commissures are resuspended inside the graft and secured with horizontal mattress sutures of 4-0 polypropylene. These sutures are then used to secure the remnants

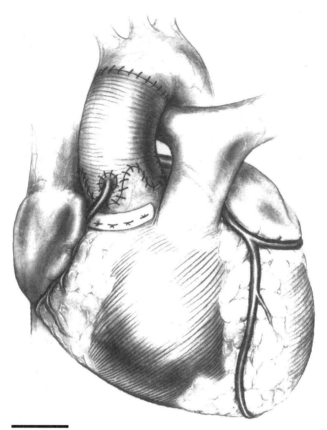

FIGURE 19.
Aortic root remodeling in patients with annuloaortic ectasia. The three
aortic sinuses are replaced as illustrated in Figures 16 and 17. Note the
Dacron band below the sinuses used to correct the dilated aortic annulus.
(Reproduced from David TE: Remodeling of the aortic root and preservation of the native aortic valve. *Op Tech Cardiac Thorac Surg* 1:44-56,
1996.)

of the aortic sinuses to the Dacron graft with a continuous in-and-
out suture line. The coronary arteries are reimplanted in their
respective sinuses.

REPAIR OF AORTIC VALVE IN AORTIC DISSECTIONS
Patients with aortic dissections may have AI because of dilatation
of the aortic root or detachment of one or more commissures of the
aortic valve, or both. If the aortic root is dilated but the leaflets are
normal, remodeling of the aortic root as described above is performed. In case of acute type A aortic dissection without aortic
root aneurysm, resuspension of the detached commissures and
replacement of the ascending aorta with a tubular Dacron graft of

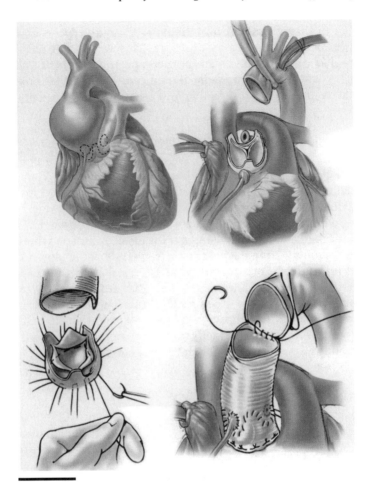

FIGURE 20.
Reimplantation of the aortic valve for aortic root aneurysm with annuloaortic ectasia. Multiple sutures are placed all around the left ventricular outflow tract and then through a tailored Dacron graft. The aortic valve is placed inside of the graft and the sutures are tied on the outside. The three commissures are resuspended in the Dacron graft, and the remnants of the sinuses wall are sutured to the graft. The coronary arteries are reimplanted in their respective new sinuses.

appropriate diameter sutured right at the sinotubular junction restores normal aortic valve function. In cases of extensive dissection of the aortic sinuses, reimplantation of the aortic valve is an ideal operative procedure because all dissected tissues are excised and the aortic valve is secured within a tubular Dacron graft as described above. This technique is associated with a very low risk of bleeding along the proximal suture line in comparison with the remodeling procedure.

Ten to fifteen percent of patients with acute type A aortic dissection have a bicuspid aortic valve. This valve does not need to be replaced if the leaflets are normal and the root is not aneurysmal. However, if the root is dilated, we believe that composite replacement of the aortic valve and ascending aorta is better than a valve-sparing procedure.

SUBAORTIC MEMBRANEOUS VENTRICULAR SEPTAL DEFECT

Subaortic membraneous ventricular septal defect is a congenital lesion that is often associated with prolapse of the right aortic leaflet and AI. Most surgeons repair the aortic valve by closing the ventricular septal defect with a patch and by plicating the free margin of the prolapsing right aortic leaflet.[7] Yacoub et al.[8] recently described a technique using a transaortic approach whereby the subaortic membraneous ventricular septal defect is closed primarily with multiple mattressed sutures passed from the crest of the ventricular septum through the aortic annulus and into the thinned portion of the sinus of Valsalva. These stitches are supposed to elevate the aortic annulus of the right aortic leaflet and correct the AI. If this maneuver does not correct the leaflet prolapse entirely because the leaflet has become elongated, plication of the free margin is added.

RHEUMATIC AORTIC INSUFFICIENCY

Repair of the aortic valve in patients with rheumatic disease and severe AI is usually not feasible without leaflet augmentation with glutaraldehyde-fixed autologous or bovine pericardium.[9] Rheumatic patients who need mitral valve surgery and have mild or moderate AI sometimes have enough leaflet tissue to correct AI without leaflet augmentation. Commissurotomy, shaving the leaflets to make them thinner and more pliable, plication of the subcommissural triangles, and reduction of the diameter of the sinotubular junction are maneuvers used in these cases.

DISCUSSION

The single most important determinant of feasibility of aortic valve repair is the quality of the aortic valve leaflets. There must be enough leaflet tissue of good quality to satisfactorily restore normal valve function. Luckily, dilatation of the aortic root is a common cause of AI, and the leaflets are normal or have minimal pathologic changes. The AI is caused by dilatation of the sinotubular junction, and most patients have an ascending aortic aneurysm or mega-aorta syndrome. If the sinuses of Valsalva are not excessively dilated, all that is needed to reestablish valve competence is to correct the diameter of the sinotubular junction. If the diameter of the aortic sinuses exceeds 40 mm, they should be replaced. When the entire aortic root is dilated including the aortic annulus, such as in Marfan syndrome, a more complicated operative procedure is necessary to correct AI and prevent further annular dilatation. An aortic annuloplasty should be added to the aortic root remodeling procedure. Alternatively, the aortic valve can be reimplanted inside a tubular Dacron conduit. A review of our experience with aortic valve–sparing operations in patients with aortic root aneurysms was recently published.[10] From May 1988 to December 1997, 126 patients with ascending aorta and/or aortic root aneurysm and AI underwent replacement of the ascending aorta and reconstruction of the aortic root with preservation of the native aortic valve. There were 85 men and 41 women with a mean age of 54 years (range, 14-84 years). Thirty-two patients had Marfan syndrome, 17 patients had acute and 10 patients had chronic type A aortic dissection, 23 had transverse aortic arch aneurysm, 26 had coronary artery disease, and 8 had mitral insufficiency. The aortic valve repair consisted of simple adjustment of the sinotubular junction in 33 patients, remodeling of the aortic root with replacement of one or more aortic sinuses in 60, and reimplantation of the aortic valve in a tubular Dacron graft in 33 patients. Fifteen patients also had prolapse of one aortic leaflet that was repaired with Gore-Tex sutures. There were 3 operative deaths caused by cardiac failure. Patients were followed up from 2 to 117 months (mean 31 months). There were 11 late deaths: 7 cardiovascular and 4 noncardiovascular. The actuarial survival was 72% at 7 years; it was 100% for the patients with Marfan syndrome. The freedom from reoperation for severe AI was 97% at 7 years. Only 3 patients have moderate AI; the remaining patients have mild, trace, or no AI. There have been no differences in the outcomes of patients who had remodeling of the aortic root or reimplantation of the aortic valve during our first decade of experience with these procedures.

Yacoub et al.[11] recently published their late results with aortic root remodeling in 158 patients with ascending aortic aneurysms and AI, including 68 with Marfan syndrome. The actuarial survival at 10 years was approximately 80%, and the freedom from reoperation was 89%. Schafers et al.[12] compared the results of remodeling of the aortic root with those of reimplantation of the aortic valve in patients with aortic root aneurysm and found similar clinical and echocardiographic outcome.

Some investigators have expressed concerns regarding the appropriateness of preserving the aortic valve in patients with Marfan syndrome because they have abnormal fibrillin.[13,14] However, ours and Yacoub's experiences suggest that aortic valve repair in these patients is durable.[10,11] Patients with myxomatous mitral valve also have abnormal fibrillin in the leaflets.[14] The experience with mitral valve repair in these patients indicates that recurrence of the prolapse is rare during the first decade of follow-up.[15] By analogy, stabilization of the aortic annulus and sinotubular junction with a properly tailored Dacron graft may prevent or retard degenerative changes of the connective tissue of the aortic leaflets.

Cosgrove et al.[16] showed that incompetent bicuspid aortic valves could be satisfactorily repaired by a triangular resection of the leaflet with prolapse, resection of the raphe, and plication of the subcommissural triangles if the annulus was dilated. The group from the Cleveland Clinic have accumulated a sizeable experience with repair of incompetent bicuspid aortic valves, and recently reported their experience with 94 patients.[17,18] Most of their patients were men (93%), with a mean age of 38 years. The freedom from reoperation was 84% at 7 years. The only predictive factor for reoperation was residual AI after the repair. There were no operative or late deaths in that series.[17]

Our experience with repair of bicuspid aortic valves with AI caused by prolapse of one leaflet is limited to 22 patients during the past 5 years. In 19 patients, the repair consisted of a triangular resection or plication of the central portion of the prolapsing leaflet in all patients and plication of the subcommissural triangles in 6 patients. Three patients had nonprolapsing leaflets, and the AI was caused by dilatation of the sinotubular junction and ascending aortic aneurysm. These 3 patients had a remodeling procedure. There has been only one failure resulting from leaflet prolapse in a patient who had remodeling of the aortic root. None of the other 21 patients have more than mild AI, and it seems stable. Thus, patients with bicuspid aortic valve and AI resulting from prolapse of one leaflet without aortic root aneurysm appear to do well after aortic valve repair.[19]

Resuspension of detached commissures during repair of acute type A aortic dissection has provided good long-term results in most patients.[20,21] We believe that recurrent AI in those patients is usually caused by dilatation of the aortic root. Thus, if the root is dilated but the leaflets are fairly normal, simple resuspension of the commissures is doomed to fail because the root will continue to dilate. These patients should have remodeling of the aortic root or reimplantation of the aortic valve. We believe that reimplantation of the aortic valve is ideal for patients with acute type A aortic dissection and dilated root because it is associated with lower risk of bleeding along the proximal suture line.

Congenital subaortic ventricular septal defect is frequently associated with prolapse of the right coronary cusp and AI.[7,8,22]

Patients with this lesion are often operated on before reaching adulthood. Most surgeons have used the technique of closing the ventricular septal defect with a patch and plicating the free margin of the right cusp to correct its prolapse.[7,22] Trusler et al.[7] reported a freedom from aortic valve replacement of 85% at 10 years using the above technique. Yacoub et al.[8] recently reported a new approach to this syndrome whereby the septal defect is closed primarily with the same sutures used to remodel the aortic annulus and dilated sinus of Valsalva. These investigators described 46 patients with this syndrome. During a mean follow-up of 8.4 years, only 5 patients required aortic valve replacement.

Aortic valve repair for AI caused by rheumatic disease is seldom feasible because the leaflets are often fibrotic, thickened, and fused. Thus, patients with advanced rheumatic changes in the aortic valve are not candidates for aortic valve repair. Repair of these valves requires leaflet augmentation with glutaraldehyde-fixed autologous or heterologous pericardium.[9] This operative procedure has been performed since the early days of cardiac surgery.[23] This technique has been used largely in young rheumatic patients, but most reports give only short-term results.[9]

The only rheumatic aortic valves we have repaired are in patients who need mitral valve surgery and have moderate AI. At surgery, the leaflets are found to be mildly fibrotic but still pliable. We have on occasion shaved them to increase their pliability, but more often we simply plicate the subcommissural triangles and sinotubular junction to increase leaflet coaptation. These maneuvers seem to reduce or eliminate AI in patients with mild or moderate rheumatic involvement of the aortic valve. However, the long-term results appear to be disappointing according to a recent report by Bernal et al.[24] These investigators followed up a group of 55 patients who had aortic valve repair for mild or moderate rheumatic aortic valve disease at the time of mitral valve surgery for almost two decades. The freedom from aortic valve deterioration at 20 years was 25%.

We believe that aortic valve repair for AI should be reserved for straightforward cases with normal or minimally diseased leaflets, in which the mechanism of AI results from leaflet prolapse, dilatation of the sinotubular junction, or dilatation of the aortic annulus. Aortic valve repair should also be performed in patients with bicuspid aortic valves with minimally dilated aortic roots in whom AI is caused by prolapse of only one of the two leaflets. Patients with degenerative disease of the aortic valve with overstretched, thinned, and prolapsing leaflets and those with rheumatic disease with fibrotic and fused leaflets are better served with aortic valve replacement.

REFERENCES

1. Kunzelman KS, Grande J, David TE, et al: Aortic root and valve relationships. Impact on surgical repair. *J Thorac Cardiovasc Surg* 107:162-170, 1994.
2. Sadee A, Becker AE, Verheul HA, et al: Aortic valve regurgitation and the congenitally bicuspid aortic valve: A clinico-pathological correlation. *Br Heart J* 67:439-441, 1992.
3. Edwards WD, Leaf DS, Edwards JE: Dissecting aortic aneurysm associated with congenital bicuspid aortic valve. *Circulation* 57:1022-1025, 1978.
4. Olson LJ, Subramanian R, Edwards WD: Surgical pathology of pure aortic insufficiency: A study of 225 cases. *Mayo Clin Proc* 59:835-841, 1984.
5. David TE, Feindel CM, Bos J: Repair of the aortic valve in patients with aortic insufficiency and aortic root aneurysm. *J Thorac Cardiovasc Surg* 109:345-352, 1995.
6. David TE: Remodeling of the aortic root and preservation of the native aortic valve. *Op Tech Cardiac Thorac Surg* 1:44-56, 1996.
7. Trusler GA, Williams WG, Smallhorn JF, et al: Late results after repair of aortic insufficiency associated with ventricular septal defect. *J Thorac Cardivoasc Surg* 103:276-281, 1992.
8. Yacoub MH, Khan H, Stavri G, et al: Anatomic correction of the syndrome of prolapsing right coronary aortic cusp, dilatation of the sinus of Valsalva, and ventricular septal defect. *J Thorac Cardiovasc Surg* 113:253-260, 1998.
9. Duran CMG: Aortic valve repair and reconstruction. *Op Tech Cardiac Thorac Surg* 1:15-29, 1996.
10. David TE: Aortic valve sparing operations: An update. *Ann Thorac Surg,* in press.
11. Yacoub MH, Gehle P, Chandrasekaran V, et al: Late results of a valve-preserving operation in patients with aneurysms of the ascending aorta and root. *J Thorac Cardiovasc Surg* 115:1080-1090, 1998.
12. Schafers HJ, Fries R, Langer F, et al: Valve-preserving replacement of the ascending aorta: Remodeling versus reimplantation. *J Thorac Cardiovasc Surg* 116:990-996, 1998.
13. Gott VL, Laschinger JC, Cameron DE, et al: The Marfan syndrome and the cardiovascular surgeon. *Eur J Cardiothorac Surg* 10:149-158, 1996.
14. Nousari HC, Fleischer KJ, Anhalt GJ, et al: Demonstration of fibrillin abnormalities in cardiovascular tissue of patients with Marfan's syndrome. *Circulation* 92(Suppl 1):442A, 1995.
15. David TE, Omran A, Armstrong S, et al: Long-term results of mitral valve repair for myxomatous disease with and without chordal replacement with expanded polytetrafluoroethylene sutures. *J Thorac Cardiovasc Surg* 115:1279-1286, 1998.
16. Cosgrove DM, Rosenkranz ER, Hendren WG, et al: Valvuloplasty for aortic insufficiency. *J Thorac Cardiovasc Surg* 102:571-577, 1991.
17. Fraser CD Jr, Wang N, Mee RBB, et al: Repair of insufficient bicuspid aortic valves. *Ann Thorac Surg* 58:386-390, 1994.
18. Casselman FP, Gillinov AM, Akhrass R, et al: Intermediate-term dura-

bility of bicuspid aortic valve repair for prolapsing leaflet. *Eur J Cardiothorac Surg* 15:302-308, 1999.

19. Moidl R, Moritz A, Simon P, et al: Echocardiographic results after repair of incompetent bicuspid aortic valves. *Ann Thorac Surg* 60:669-672, 1995.

20. Fann JI, Glower DD, Miller DC, et al: Preservation of the aortic valve in type A aortic dissection complicated by aortic regurgitation. *J Thorac Cardiovasc Surg* 102:62-73, 1991.

21. Mazzucotelli JP, Deleuze PH, Baufreton C, et al: Preservation of the aortic valve in acute aortic dissection: Long-term echocardiographic assessment and clinical outcome. *Ann Thorac Surg* 55:1513-1517, 1993.

22. Chavaud S, Serraf A, Mihaileanu S, et al: Ventricular septal defect associated with aortic valve incompetence: Results of two surgical management. Ann Thorac Surg 1990;49:875-880.

23. Bailey CP: Valvular heart disease: The reconstructive approach, in Davila JC (ed): *Second Henry Ford Hospital International Symposium on Cardiac Surgery.* New York, Appleton-Century-Crofts, 1977, pp 7-29.

24. Bernal JM, Fernandez-Vales M, Rabasa JM, et al: Repair of non-severe rheumatic aortic valve disease during other valvular procedures: Is it safe? *J Thorac Cardiovasc Surg* 115:1130-1135, 1998.

CHAPTER 7

Scimitar Syndrome

Charles B. Huddleston, M.D.
Associate Professor of Surgery, Division of Cardiothoracic Surgery,
Department of Surgery, Washington University School of Medicine;
Chief, Pediatric Cardiothoracic Surgery, St. Louis Children's Hospital,
St. Louis, Missouri

Eric N. Mendeloff, M.D.
Assistant Professor of Surgery, Division of Cardiothoracic Surgery,
Department of Surgery, Washington University School of Medicine;
Attending Pediatric Cardiothoracic Surgeon, St. Louis Children's
Hospital, St. Louis, Missouri

Scimitar syndrome is a rare congenital malformation occurring in approximately 1 to 3 of every 100,000 live births.[1] The most characteristic finding of this syndrome is partial anomalous pulmonary venous drainage of all or part of the right lung to the inferior vena cava (IVC). The anomalously draining right pulmonary vein courses in a crescentic fashion along the right heart border, eventually curving sharply to the left as it approaches the diaphragm to enter the IVC. The name of the syndrome derives from the observation that on an anterior chest radiograph, this vein will cast an image reminiscent of a Turkish sword, or *scimitar* (Fig 1). This rarest form of partial anomalous pulmonary venous return rarely occurs as an isolated lesion because there is variable association with hypoplasia of the right lung, bronchial anomalies, dextroposition or dextrorotation of the heart, hypoplasia of the right pulmonary artery, and anomalous systemic arterial supply to the lower lobe of the right lung (Fig 2). Additionally, there may be a variety of associated congenital heart defects ranging from relatively common lesions such as a secundum atrial septal defect or a patent ductus arteriosus to more complex entities such as tetralogy of Fallot or truncus arteriosus.

Because this syndrome has become more recognized in recent years, there has been a tendency to delineate patients with this

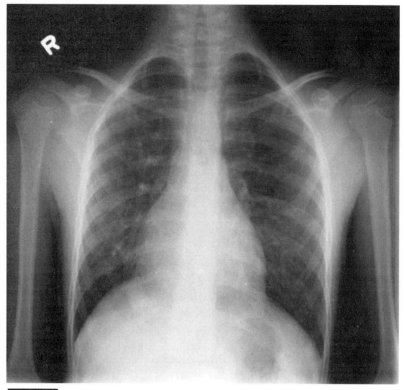

FIGURE 1.
Frontal chest x-ray from a 13-year-old patient with scimitar syndrome. One can faintly note the curvilinear density parallel to the right heart border descending to a point below the diaphragm—the scimitar sign. *Abbreviation: R,* right side.

entity into two major categories: an infantile form and a pediatric or adult form. This differentiation is based more on the pathophysiologic impact and clinical presentation than on an actual difference in anatomic substrate. As will be further described in this chapter, the infantile form tends to have a greater association with complex cardiovascular anomalies and carries a worse prognosis than the pediatric or adult variant.

HISTORY

Given the rarity of the lesion, it is perhaps a bit unusual that the first pathologic descriptions of what would eventually come to be called scimitar syndrome came in 1836 from two separate investigators in different countries, Chassinat in France and Cooper in England.[2,3] It wasn't until 1949 that Dotter et al.[4] used angiocar-

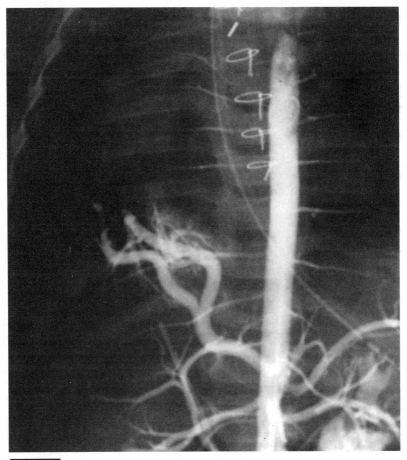

FIGURE 2.
The anomalous systemic arterial supply arising from the abdominal aorta and ascending through the diaphragm to supply a large portion of the right lower lobe.

diography to report the first two cases in the literature in which partial anomalous pulmonary venous return of the right lung to the IVC was diagnosed premortem and nonsurgically. The groundwork for what would eventually come to be an important part of the surgical therapy for this disease came in 1950 when Gerbode and Hultgren published their experimental observations on performance of atriovenous anastomoses.[5] Based on technical insights stemming from Gerbode's work, as well as the success obtained by Gross and Watkins,[6] Kirklin et al.[7] would perform the first successful attempt at physiologic repair of partial anomalous pulmonary venous return of the right lung to the IVC associated with an atrial septal defect. This repair was on a 32-year-old housewife and was performed by disconnecting the pulmonary venous trunk from where it entered the IVC below the diaphragm and reimplanting it on the posterior wall of the right atrium opposite the atrial septal defect. Then, using the atrio-septo-pexy of Bailey et al.[8] and a synthetic patch, the atrial septal defect was closed in such a fashion that the pulmonary venous flow from the right lung was directed across the defect into the left atrium. Kirklin et al. emphasized the importance of occluding the inflow into the right lung during this procedure.

The same year that Kirklin published his surgical success with this entity, Halasz et al.[9] appear to have been the first to mention the similarity in shape on frontal chest radiograph of the anomalously draining pulmonary vein to a scimitar. Under the section on radiographic findings, Halasz et al. note "...in the plain films the most striking appearance, which should at once suggest the diagnosis, was that of a dagger or scimitar-shaped vascular density more or less parallel to the right cardiac border..."

Finally, it was Neill et al.[10] in 1960 who, in focusing on a case of familial occurrence of hypoplastic lung with systemic arterial supply and venous drainage, coined the term *scimitar syndrome*. Up until 1960, there were only 35 cases reported in the literature, and it wasn't until 1973 that Kuiper-Oosterwal and Moulaert[11] reported the first two cases of scimitar syndrome diagnosed in infants before 2 months of age. Since then, there have been several series reported that have helped to delineate the spectrum, natural history, and best forms of therapy for this malformation.

EMBRYOLOGY

Scimitar syndrome is a unique combination of anomalies having no unifying explanation. In this regard, the salient features deserving repetition include hypoplasia of the right lung, anomalous pulmonary venous drainage from all or part of the right lung, systemic arterial supply to a portion of the right lower lobe that does not correlate with the venous effluent draining anomalously, and the consistency of the right-sided nature of the anomaly—there have been only two reported cases of scimitar syndrome involving the left lung.[12,13] In the normal sequence of events, major branches of the peripheral pulmonary veins form a common pulmonary vein which then merges into the dorsal surface of the atrium during the sixth gestational week.[14] Anomalous pulmonary venous drainage results from the failure of part or all of the pulmonary venous system to orient properly toward the atrium. The affected pulmonary veins then drain via persisting extrapulmonary communications.

The pulmonary arteries develop from the sixth aortic arch. However, the earliest arterial supply to the primitive lung is via the primordial postbranchial plexus of the descending thoracic aorta. Normally this group of vessels persists as bronchial arteries.[15] If there is incomplete development of the pulmonary arterial system, this anomalous systemic arterial supply may represent an orderly substitution from the dorsal aorta for vessels normally derived in continuity with the more proximal sixth aortic arch.

Although there are similarities between scimitar syndrome and pulmonary sequestration, the major difference is that all parts of the lung are connected to the central tracheobronchial tree in cases of scimitar syndrome.[16] In addition, in true pulmonary sequestration, the affected portion of lung supplied by a systemic artery is that portion with venous drainage to the systemic venous system.

ASSOCIATED PULMONARY ANOMALIES

The most obvious pulmonary abnormalities associated with scimitar syndrome are the hypoplastic nature of the right lung and the compensatory growth of the left lung. Apart from the large size of the left lung, there are no other significant abnormalities involving the disorder. There may be an incomplete pleural envelope for the right lung or none at all. The lobation of the right lung is also frequently abnormal by external exam; there may be one, two, or three lobes. The middle lobe is the one most frequently absent. The bronchial branching pattern is also frequently abnormal and may present as a mirror image of the left lung. The right upper lobe may be hyparterial (arising from underneath the pulmonary artery), as opposed to its usual pattern. All parts of the right lung connect to the central tracheobronchial tree.[16] However, there may be diverticula or cystic changes of the bronchi. These cystic bronchial changes may be the source of infections in older patients.[9] So-called "horseshoe lung" has been reported in association with scimitar syndrome. In this entity, there is fusion between the posteroinferior portions of the right and left lungs behind the heart and in front of the esophagus. This has no significant pathologic significance by itself, except that a pneumothorax could be bilateral, should it occur.[17] The lung parenchyma itself seems to be normal.

The arterial supply to the right lung is derived from three sources: the right pulmonary artery, the bronchial artery, and the abnormal systemic artery (or arteries) from the thoracic, abdominal, or diaphragmatic vessels. The right pulmonary artery is frequently hypoplastic and occasionally absent. The bronchial artery arises from the proximal descending thoracic aorta and supplies the bronchi in the usual fashion. The abnormal systemic arteries are usually derived from the abdominal aorta but may arise from the thoracic aorta. There might be multiple arteries, but more common-ly this arterial supply occurs as a single vessel penetrating the diaphragm and reaching the right lower lobe by way of the inferior pulmonary ligament. It has frequently branched while traversing the inferior pulmonary ligament, giving the impression of the involve-ment of multiple vessels. It is unclear whether the subsequent branching course of these vessels is more like a pulmonary or bronchial artery; however, after careful examination, a pattern more typical of the pulmonary artery can be found. Some patients have developed histologic changes suggestive of pulmonary hypertension in the region of the lung supplied by these anomalous arteries.[9]

The anomalous pulmonary vein representing the *sine qua non* of this syndrome may be the pulmonary venous drainage for all or part of the right lung. In approximately two thirds of cases it is the sole venous drainage of the right lung; in the others, there are vari-able amounts connecting in the normal fashion to the left atrium. The anomalous vein's descent in the chest parallels the right heart border, and as it receives tributaries from the lung it gradually enlarges. In most instances it joins the IVC below the diaphragm, but it may also join the systemic venous return at the inferior cavoatrial junction or at the inferior portion of the right atrium.[18] The orifice of this vein frequently appears slightly smaller than the largest portion of the body of the vein. Clearly defined stenosis of the vein occurs in about 10% of patients; some of those will also have stenosis in the pulmonary veins on the left. This is a partic-ularly lethal problem. In rare cases there may be two of these veins descending next to each other in the chest.

PRESENTATION IN INFANCY
CLINICAL PRESENTATION
Unlike older children and teenagers with scimitar syndrome, infants requiring medical attention for treatment of this disorder are frequently quite symptomatic. Symptoms, such as tachypnea and poor weight gain, are generally due to heart failure. Some have cyanosis. The definition of the infantile presentation of this syn-drome is arbitrarily defined as presentation during the first year of life. However, most infants who do become symptomatic do so by 2 months of age. Combining the series from The Hospital for Sick Children in Toronto[19] and from 12 European centers[20] with our own findings, we determine that 70% of these infants were brought in within 60 days of birth. Virtually all had what were described as "severe" symptoms. In some cases, associated lesions, such as a ventricular septal defect, appear to have contributed to the early appearance of heart failure. However, that was not true in all instances. Why some infants develop severe symptoms with

anatomic lesions similar to those seen in asymptomatic teenagers is unclear. Pulmonary hypertension is almost always present in these infants, however. The chest radiograph typically shows dextroposition of the cardiac silhouette and a hypoplastic right lung. The scimitar sign from which the name of this syndrome is derived is ordinarily not present, being frequently hidden by the right heart border and the thymic shadow. Thus, an infant with tachypnea and a chest x-ray showing a small right lung should be suspected of having scimitar syndrome. In a review of 33 patients with underdevelopment of 1 lung, scimitar syndrome was present in 8, the others having a variety of other problems including accessory diaphragm, small diaphragmatic hernia, simple hypoplasia of the lung, and congenital absence of the pulmonary artery.[21]

ASSOCIATED LESIONS

An atrial septal defect (or *patent foramen ovale*) is frequently present in patients with scimitar syndrome. Approximately half of all these infants with this defect have a patent ductus arteriosus as well. One third will have more complex associated cardiac lesions, such as ventricular septal defects, coarctation of the aorta, or tetralogy of Fallot. In most patients, an abnormal systemic artery originating from the abdominal aorta supplies all or part of the right lower lobe. Pulmonary hypertension is extremely common in these infants, even those in which an atrial septal defect is the only other associated lesion. The etiology of the pulmonary hypertension is frequently related to the associated lesions, which include a ventricular septal defect or stenosis of the pulmonary venous drainage. However, in those with only an associated atrial septal defect, the cause is unclear. The systemic artery supplying a portion of the right lung may play a role in this by producing a significant left-to-right shunt through a relatively small lung. Another, perhaps more plausible, theory is that there is failure of the pulmonary circulation to adapt normally following birth in the presence of the left-to-right shunt.[22]

CARDIAC CATHETERIZATION

A cardiac catheterization should always be performed to document the diagnosis, to identify the specific nature of the pulmonary venous drainage, to examine for the presence of pulmonary hypertension and possible pulmonary venous stenosis, and to evaluate for other associated cardiac lesions. Pulmonary hypertension is nearly always present, as mentioned above. Every effort should be made to identify the anomalous systemic arterial supply to the right lung. Coil embolization of the systemic arterial collaterals can be performed in this setting. Although concerns

TABLE 1.

Combined Series From Toronto, Europe, and St. Louis

	Patients	Overall Mortality	Medical Therapy	Occlusion of Anom Sys Artery	PDA ligation/ CoA repair	Complete Repair	Pulm Resection
Toronto	19	5	7 (1)	5 (3)	2 (2)	6 (0)	1 (0)
Europe	25	16	10 (7)	6 (1)	5 (5)	0 (0)	3 (2)
St. Louis	12	4	2 (2)	1 (1)	0 (0)	7 (1)	2 (0)
Total	56	24 (45%)	19 (10)	12 (5)	7 (7)	13 (1)*	6 (2)†

Note: This is a compilation of the infants from 3 large series: The Hospital for Sick Children in Toronto, a consortium of centers in Europe, and from our own series at St. Louis Children's Hospital. Numbers in parentheses indicate the absolute number of deaths for each treatment category, except when indicated as percentage.

*Reoperations following repair: lung transplant (2), pneumonectomy (3), repair of pulmonary vein stenosis (1).

†Three other patients required right pneumonectomy because of failed repair.

Abbreviations: Anom, anomalous; *Sys,* systemic; *PDA,* patent ductus arteriosus; *CoA,* coarctation of the aorta; *Pulm,* pulmonary.

have been raised about the risk of infarction of the lung with this procedure, to date there have been no reports of this complication.

TREATMENT

Table 1 summarizes the results of treatment from the three largest series in the literature. It comprises a total of 56 patients from The Hospital for Sick Children in Toronto,[19] a consortium of centers in Europe,[20] and our own series at St. Louis Children's Hospital. The overall mortality of all infants (who were treated in a variety of ways) was 45%. This obviously speaks to the lethality of this lesion when symptoms occur during the first year of life.

Medical Therapy

A trial of medical therapy is a reasonable initial approach for very young infants to increase their size before repair of the defect. However, the presence of pulmonary hypertension is a poor prognostic sign. Failure to respond to medical therapy or the persistence of pulmonary hypertension demands proceeding on to surgery. The mortality with medical therapy alone from the combined series in Table 1 is 53%.

Surgical Therapy

When it comes to which approach to take for operative intervention, there are many options. Information from the literature is clouded by relatively small series of patients covering many years, a diversity of approaches in each individual series, multiple operations performed on the same patient, and different associated anomalies that, independently, have an impact on the prognosis. We can see from Table 1 that ligation of the patent ductus arteriosus or repair of coarctation of the aorta alone has a high mortality. Many have such severe elevation of the pulmonary vascular resistance that the degree of shunting across the ductus is small or even net right to left.[19] Ligation of the anomalous systemic arterial supply to the right lung has had mixed results. Some have reported excellent results when this is the sole form of therapy for these infants.[20,23] Coil embolization performed as part of a cardiac catheterization effectively does the same thing,[24,25] and, as mentioned above, this ought to be a part of the routine cardiac catheterization when performed as the initial diagnostic procedure. Those patients categorized in Table 1 as having occlusion of the anomalous systemic artery underwent either surgical or catheter occlusion of these vessels. Obviously there are some infants who benefitted from this as their sole form of therapy. However, our experience (and that of others[19]) with this alone has not been rewarding because there has been persistence of either heart failure or pulmonary hypertension resulting in death or the need to proceed with repair.

Ideally, repair of this lesion would consist of a redirection of the anomalous pulmonary venous drainage, occlusion of the anomalous systemic arteries, and repair of all associated cardiac lesions. The initial technique described for repair of the anomalous pulmonary venous drainage entailed a long baffle from the entry point of the pulmonary vein into the IVC to the left atrium via an atrial septal defect (Fig 3).[23] Pulmonary venous blood thus travels in an inferior direction and then turns nearly 180 degrees to run superiorly toward the atrial septal defect. Deep hypothermia and circulatory arrest are necessary to accurately place this baffle around the orifice of the anomalous pulmonary veins and to avoid the entry points of the nearby hepatic veins in these small infants. In addition, cannulation of the IVC is extremely difficult due to the proximity of the hepatic veins and the caudad location of the orifice of the anomalous pulmonary veins. This technique has worked reasonably well in older children and adults, but an important shortcoming is its inability to address stenosis at the orifice of the pulmonary vein. In infants there has been a high failure rate due to stenosis or obstruction in the venous drainage, either at the orifice of the pulmonary vein into the IVC or along the course of the baffle itself.[19] The baffle is generally constructed with pericardium, which is subject to thickening and contracture; in some

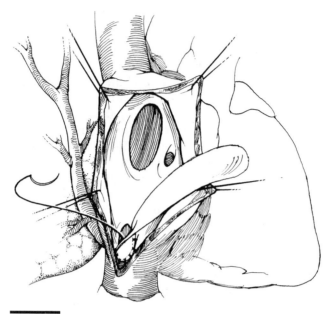

FIGURE 3.
The long intra-atrial baffle repair requires a large patch of either pericardium or synthetic material to sew around the orifice of the anomalous pulmonary vein as it enters the inferior vena cava. The rest of the baffle is created within the right atrium by sewing this patch up to and around the atrial septal defect. (Reprinted with permission from the Society of Thoracic Surgeons, from *The Annals of Thoracic Surgery*, 1999, vol. 67, in press.)

instances synthetic material can be used, but this also may become obstructed because of the development of a thick pseudointima. The IVC will also require patch enlargement to accommodate this baffle, which takes up space in the IVC. Otherwise, obstruction can develop there (Fig 4).

A better approach for infants is one in which the anomalous vein is taken off the IVC with a small segment of the wall of the IVC, mobilized superiorly, and reimplanted into the left atrium or, more commonly, the posterolateral wall of the right atrium (Fig 5). From there, the distance to the left atrium via the atrial septal defect is shorter and more direct. This reimplantation technique was first described Kirklin et al.[7] and then popularized by Shumacker and Judd.[26] The IVC should be patched, and we prefer synthetic material to avoid the propensity of pericardium to shrink. Taking a rim of IVC with the anomalous vein provides slightly more length and stronger tissue for suture and also allows for enlargement of the orifice of the vein by opening it longitudinally. The true incidence of stenosis of the orifice of this vein in

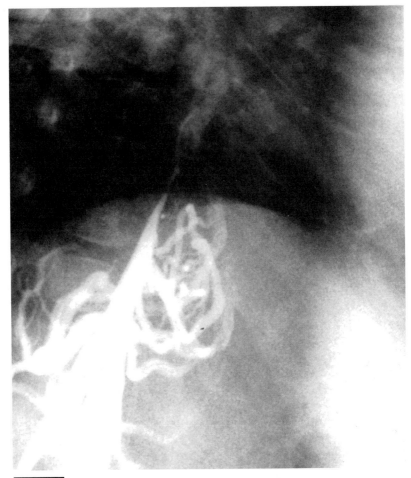

FIGURE 4.
An angiogram of the inferior vena cava in a patient treated with an intra-atrial baffle for repair of the scimitar syndrome. There is a tight stenosis of the inferior vena cava at the level of the diaphragm and extending into the right atrium.

infants is unknown, but may be very high. Frequently the entry appears angiographically smaller than the body of the vein, although the pressure gradient at this level may be either very low or zero. However, the late follow-up of infants repaired using an intra-atrial baffle as described in the previous paragraph demonstrates a high incidence of stenosis at that level.[19]

This reimplantation technique may not be appropriate for all patients. We have encountered 3 patients in whom the anomalous pulmonary vein descended the right chest in a posterior position,

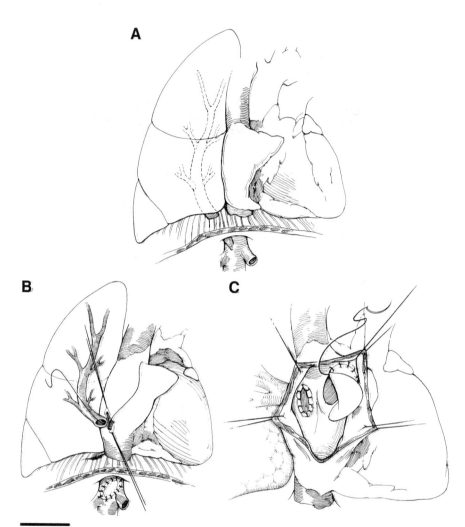

FIGURE 5.

A, course of the anomalous pulmonary venous drainage in a patient with scimitar syndrome. Note that the pulmonary vein on the right enters the inferior vena cava below the diaphragm. **B,** the pulmonary vein has been divided off the inferior vena cava and mobilized in a cephalad direction. The inferior vena cava has been patched with pericardium or synthetic material. An opening in the posterolateral wall of the right atrium has been created and the pulmonary vein is being anastomosed to that. **C,** a relatively short baffle is then created between this more proximate orifice of the anomalous pulmonary vein and the entry into the left atrium via the atrial septal defect. (Reprinted with permission from the Society of Thoracic Surgeons, from *The Annals of Thoracic Surgery*, 1999, vol. 67, in press.)

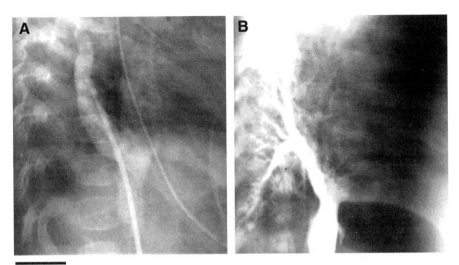

FIGURE 6.
A, frame from an angiogram; a straight lateral view of the anomalous pulmonary vein in an infant with scimitar syndrome. Note the position of the vein relative to the spine and the esophagus (marked by the presence of the nasogastric tube). The vein lies in a posterior position throughout much of its course in the chest and then moves anterior at the level of the diaphragm to enter the inferior vena cava below the diaphragm. **B**, another infant with scimitar syndrome. The angiogram of the anomalous pulmonary vein is again shown in a straight lateral projection of the chest. Note that the vein is anterior to the body of the spine well above the diaphragm before entering the inferior vena cava. (Reprinted with permission from the Society of Thoracic Surgeons, from *The Annals of Thoracic Surgery*, 1999, vol. 67, in press.)

coming anterior at the level of the diaphragm to enter the IVC below the diaphragm. Although this vein runs along the anterior surface of the hilar region of the lung in most cases (Fig 6), in those infants in which the vein runs posteriorly it is difficult to mobilize the vein sufficiently to reach the right or left atrium without kinking. Two of these infants were repaired with a long intra-atrial baffle from the orifice in the IVC to the atrial septal defect. In both cases the baffle obstructed and a pneumonectomy was required; one of these infants survived and the other died. The third infant was treated with primary right pneumonectomy and has done well. Thus, in symptomatic infants with scimitar syndrome and an anomalous pulmonary vein draining posteriorly in the right hemithorax, we recommend right pneumonectomy rather than an attempt at repair.

Potential long-term risks of a pneumonectomy performed on an infant include scoliosis, chronic respiratory insufficiency, and post-pneumonectomy syndrome. In a large series of patients undergoing pneumonectomy during early childhood years, however, the compensatory growth of the contralateral lung nearly made up for the loss. In fact, there were no obvious untoward effects in these patients followed up for more than 30 years.[27] Patients with scimitar syndrome have a right lung that is significantly smaller than a normal right lung to begin with, and the left lung has frequently already undergone compensatory growth with some mediastinal shift producing the appearance of dextrocardia. Perfusion scans in these infants demonstrate that approximately 25% of all pulmonary perfusion goes to the small right lung. Clearly some serious complications can occur later, after pneumonectomy, but the majority of children seem to tolerate this well with only mild perturbations in pulmonary function and hemodynamics occurring.[28] Of the 6 patients treated with pulmonary resection as the only form of therapy in the three series summarized in Table 1, there have been 4 long-term survivors.

The optimal treatment for these infants is still somewhat controversial. However, given our experience and review of the available literature, we would recommend initial therapy to consist of cardiac catheterization with coil embolization of the systemic collateral arterial supply to the right lung, followed by medical therapy for heart failure. If symptoms persist, repair should be carried out, and the anomalous pulmonary vein should be reimplanted into the posterolateral wall of the right atrium at a point close to the atrial septum so that the baffle to the left atrium via the atrial septal defect can be short. If the orifice of the vein is angiographically small, then it should be enlarged during the reimplantation process. If symptoms persist after occlusion of the systemic arterial collaterals in infants in whom the anomalous pulmonary vein cannot be re-implanted, a right pneumonectomy should be performed.

PRESENTATION IN OLDER CHILDREN AND ADULTS
CLINICAL PRESENTATION

Contrary to the infantile variant, symptoms in children and adults with scimitar syndrome can be relatively subtle, with the diagnosis often made incidentally.[1] The aforementioned first two cases ever diagnosed antemortem by Dotter et al.[4] using angiocardiography were in completely asymptomatic patients; a chest radiographic test performed as part of routine screening. Najm et al.[19] collected 32 cases over 20 years and found that symptoms of heart failure were present in none of the patients diagnosed after the age of 1 year as opposed to 11 of 19 patients diagnosed during infancy. Nonetheless, with careful questioning, evidence of some symptoms can be elicited in the majority of pediatric and adult patients, with a history of dyspnea and fatigue being most common. Some patients have recurrent pulmonary infections. The etiology of this is unclear but may be related to the abnormal bronchial branching pattern mentioned above. Hypoplasia of the right lung occurs in only about 25% of the older children and adults with scimitar syndrome. The chest radiograph shows the "scimitar sign" in about 70% of patients.[1]

The left-to-right shunt at the atrial level produces cardiac examination results similar to those seen in the case of an atrial septal defect: soft systolic murmur at the left upper sternal border accompanied by a fixed split second heart sound. Some patients have come in with chest pain, palpitations, and atrial fibrillation. The electrocardiographic results demonstrate either right ventricular hypertrophy or right bundle branch block in about half the patients. Review of our own experience revealed that diagnosis was prompted by the presence of symptoms in 50% of patients, and the remainder were diagnosed after auscultation of a precordial murmur or as an incidental finding on a chest x-ray ordered for unrelated reasons.

ASSOCIATED LESIONS

One explanation for the older patients with few symptoms is that fewer have associated congenital cardiac defects. The most commonly associated lesion is an atrial septal defect, and in our experience this was present in only 22% of patients; others have reported an incidence of as high as 50%.[29] Other more significant cardiac lesions are quite uncommon. Anomalous systemic arterial supply from the infradiaphragmatic aorta is also less frequent than in the infant population, occurring in about 50% of patients. These collateral vessels also tend to be smaller and presumably of less physiologic significance.

CARDIAC CATHETERIZATION

Cardiac catheterization is indicated in all of these patients to confirm the diagnosis, to measure the pulmonary artery pressures, and to quantify the degree of left-to-right shunting. In contrast to the infant age group, pulmonary hypertension is a rare finding in the older patients. The series of older children from Toronto[19] consisted of 12 patients whose average systolic pulmonary artery pressure was 21 mm Hg. The larger series from European centers[1] demonstrated normal pulmonary artery pressures in 94 out of 122 patients, with the remainder having mild elevation of the systolic pulmonary artery pressures between 30 and 50 mm Hg. The pulmonary-to-systemic flow ratio tended to be approximately 2.5:1 in these series on average.

TREATMENT

Some controversy exists as to the best approach to pediatric and adult patients with scimitar syndrome. Dupuis et al.[1] make a case for non-surgical management. Only one third of the 37 patients who underwent surgical repair in their series were considered to have a good result. Additionally, there were 4 deaths in this group. Conversely, there were no deaths in the nonsurgical group, and quality of life remained good in 93% with an average follow-up of 12 years. Neither the indications for surgery nor the technique used for repair in the surgical cohort were clear from the report. Other surgical series have provided significantly more encouraging results. Using the previously described technique of baffling the flow from the in situ pulmonary vein across an atrial septal defect into the left atrium, Najm et al.[19] had a 100% survival at 9 years of follow-up in 9 children and adults. Two of the patients repaired in this manner did eventually develop evidence of baffle stenosis. Torres and Dietl[30] performed surgical repair on 9 children and 1 adult using the technique that we advocate (reimplantation of the pulmonary vein to the posterior right atrial wall with a short baffle to direct the blood flow across and atrial septal defect into the left atrium). Survival was 100% and there were no complications or symptoms at a mean follow-up of 55 months.[30]

Pulmonary resection should be reserved for those circumstances in which there is significant destruction of the parenchyma by repeated infections. This procedure should be limited to only that portion of lung affected. However, it is not unusual for pneumonectomy to be required because of the difficult nature of anatomic definition of the right lung into lobes or segments. There are circumstances in which stenosis of the pulmonary venous drainage occurs either with or without previous correction. This may produce pulmonary hypertension, which is treatable with a pneumonectomy.

CONCLUSIONS

Scimitar syndrome is a rare developmental anomaly that has a characteristic and consistent feature of the drainage of part or all of the pulmonary venous blood flow from the right lung into the IVC. When this occurs as an isolated phenomenon, it acts much like an atrial septal defect, and there may be few symptoms. Infants with this syndrome frequently have associated anomalies such as marked hypoplasia of the right lung, large systemic-to-pulmonary arterial collaterals, and coexistent congenital heart defects. The pathophysiologic effects in these circumstances take on greater import such that there is usually significant congestive heart failure and pulmonary hypertension. Those born with noticeably less pronounced associated anomalies tend to progress through infancy and go undiagnosed until childhood or adulthood. Nonetheless, they may have symptoms related to frequent pulmonary infections.

The key to making the diagnosis is to have a high index of suspicion when any patient has a hypoplastic right lung or the appearance of a curvilinear density parallel to the right heart border on a chest x-ray. A cardiac catheterization is recommended even in asymptomatic adults to evaluate the degree of left-to-right shunting and pulmonary arterial pressures. We recommend repair if the pulmonary-to-systemic flow ratio is greater than 1.5:1 in an asymptomatic older patient. For infants, the anomalous systemic arterial vessels should be coil-occluded first, and if the patient remains symptomatic or has persistent pulmonary hypertension then repair should be performed. Pulmonary resection is a reasonable alternative to repair for symptomatic infants in whom repair is particularly difficult or for older patients with recurrent pulmonary infections.

REFERENCES

1. Dupuis C, Charaf LAC, Brevière GM, et al: The "adult" form of scimitar syndrome. *Am J Cardiol* 70:502-507, 1992.
2. Chassinat R: Observation of remarkable anatomic abnormalities of the circulatory system with congenital hernia at the liver, without producing any particular symptom during life [French]. *Arch Gen Med* 11:80-91, 1836.
3. Cooper G: Case of malformation of the thoracic viscera: Consisting of imperfect development of the right lung and transposition of the heart. *London Med Gazette* 18:600-602, 1836.
4. Dotter CT, Hardisty NM, Steinberg I: Anomalous right pulmonary vein entering the inferior vena cava: Two cases diagnosed during life by angiocardiography and cardiac catheterization. *Am J Med Sci* 218:31-86, 1949.
5. Gerbode F, Hultgren H: Observations on experimental atriovenous anastomoses with particular reference to congenital anomalies of the venous return to the heart and cyanosis. *Surgery* 28:235-244, 1950.
6. Gross RE, Watkins E: Surgical closure of atrial septal defects. *Arch Surg* 67:670-681, 1953.
7. Kirklin JW, Ellis FH, Wood EH: Treatment of anomalous pulmonary venous connections in association with interatrial communications. *Surgery* 39:389-398, 1956.
8. Bailey CP, Boulton HE, Jamison WL, et al: Atrio-septo-pexy for interatrial septal defects. *J Thorac Surg* 23:184-219, 1953.
9. Halasz NA, Halloran KH, Liebow AA: Bronchial and arterial anomalies with drainage of the right lung into the inferior vena cava. *Circulation* 14:826-846, 1956.
10. Neill CA, Ferencz C, Sabiston DC, et al: The familial occurrence of hypoplastic right lung with systemic arterial supply and venous drainage "scimitar syndrome". *Bull Hopkins Hosp* 107:1-21, 1960.
11. Kuiper-Oosterwal CH, Moulaert A: The scimitar syndrome in infancy and childhood. *Eur J Cardiol* 1:55-61, 1973.
12. Mardini MK, Sakati NA, Lewall, DB, et al: Scimitar syndrome. *Clin Pediatr (Phila)* 21:350-354, 1982.

13. D'Cruz LA, Arcilla RA: Anomalous venous drainage of the left lung into the inferior vena cava: A case report. *Am Heart J* 67:539-544, 1964.

14. Brown AJ: The development of the pulmonary vein in the domestic cat. *Anat Rec* 7:299, 1913.

15. Huntington GS: The morphology of the pulmonary artery in the mammalia. *Anat Rec* 17:165, 1919.

16. Kiely B, Filler J, Stone S, et al: Syndrome of anomalous venous drainage of the right lung to the inferior vena cava: A review of 67 reported cases and three new cases in children. *Am J Cardiol* 20:102-116, 1967.

17. Dupuis C, Rémy J, Rémy-Jardin M, et al: The "horseshoe" lung: Six new cases. *Pediatr Pulmonol* 17:124-130, 1994.

18. Mathy J, Galey JJ, Logeais Y, et al: Anomalous pulmonary venous return into inferior vena cava and associated bronchovascular anomalies (the scimitar syndrome): Report of three cases and review of the literature. *Thorax* 23:398-407, 1968.

19. Najm HK, Williams WG, Coles JG, et al: Scimitar syndrome: Twenty years' experience and results of repair. *J Thorac Cardiovasc Surg* 112:1161-1169, 1996.

20. Dupuis C, Charaf LAC, Brevière G-M, et al: "Infantile" form of the scimitar syndrome with pulmonary hypertension. *Am J Cardiol* 71:1326-1330, 1993.

21. Currarino G, Williams B: Causes of congenital unilateral pulmonary hypoplasia: A study of 33 cases. *Pediatr Radiol* 15:15-24, 1985.

22. Haworth SG, Sauer U, Bühlmeyer K: Pulmonary hypertension in scimitar syndrome in infancy. *Br Heart J* 50:182-189, 1983.

23. Murphy JW, Kerr AR, Kirklin JW: Intracardiac repair for anomalous pulmonary venous connection of the right lung to inferior vena cava. *Ann Thor Surg* 11:38-42, 1971.

24. Dickinson DF, Galloway RW, Massey R, et al: Scimitar syndrome in infancy: Role of embolisation of systemic arterial supply to right lung. *Br Heart J* 47:468-472, 1982.

25. Pfammatter J-P, Luhmer I, Kallfelz HC: Infantile scimitar syndrome with severe pulmonary hypertension: Successful treatment with coil embolization of the systemic arterial supply to the sequestered lung. *Cardiol in the Young* 7:454-457, 1997.

26. Shumacker HB Jr, Judd D: Partial anomalous pulmonary venous return with reference to drainage into the inferior vena cava and to an intact atrial septum. *J Cardiovasc Surg* 5:271-278, 1964.

27. Laros CD, Westermann CJJ: Dilatation, compensatory growth, or both after pneumonectomy during childhood and adolescence: A thirty-year follow-up study. *J Thorac Cardiovasc Surg* 93:570-576, 1987.

28. Stiles QR, Meyer BW, Lindesmith GG, et al: The effects of pneumonectomy in children. *J Thorac Cardiovasc Surg* 58:394-400, 1969.

29. Honey M: Anomalous pulmonary venous drainage of the right lung to the inferior vena cava ("scimitar syndrome"): Clinical spectrum in older patients and role of surgery. *Q J Med* 46:463-483, 1977.

30. Torres AR, Dietl CA: Surgical management of the scimitar syndrome: An age-dependent spectrum. *Cardiovasc Surg* 1:432-438, 1993.

CHAPTER 8

Staged Surgical Approach to Neonates With Aortic Obstruction and Single Ventricle Pathophysiology

Jonah Odim, M.D., Ph.D., F.R.C.S.(C.)
Division of Cardiothoracic Surgery, UCLA School of Medicine, UCLA Medical Center, Los Angeles, California

Hillel Laks, M.D.
Professor and Chief, Division of Cardiothoracic Surgery; Director, Heart and Heart-Lung Transplant Program, UCLA Medical Center, Los Angeles, California

At present, the definitive palliation for children with a functional single ventricle is a Fontan procedure. Attaining this goal with minimum morbidity and mortality requires staged surgical interventions from birth designed to control pulmonary blood flow and pressure while preserving ventricular function and compliance. These end points and the normal diminishing pulmonary vascular resistance in the postnatal period ultimately permit successful Fontan hemodynamics minus the services of a muscular pump for the pulmonary circulation.

The neonate with a single ventricle and aortic arch obstruction, other than hypoplastic left heart syndrome, poses a uniquely difficult challenge because of (1) the stimulus for myocardial hypertrophy and failure from impedance to systemic outflow, and (2) pulmonary vascular disease from pulmonary overcirculation. In tricuspid atresia and double-inlet left ventricle (DILV) with ventriculo-arterial discordance, the muscular bulboventricular foramen (BVF) presents yet another potential site of obstruction (subaortic) between the functional single ventricular pump and the systemic circulation. The regulation of pulmonary blood flow and pressure by banding the pulmonary artery (PAB) in this setting narrows the BVF acutely, by volume unloading, and chronically, by muscular hypertrophy induced by the band. The ventricular hypertrophy caused by persistent obstruction of the systemic pathway alters diastolic function that may adversely affect long-term outcome.

A number of approaches have emerged to avoid subaortic stenosis, ventricular dysfunction, and the morbidity associated historically with PAB. These strategies include an initial modified Norwood procedure with circulatory arrest or an aortopulmonary connection (Damus-Kaye-Stansel [DKS]) on cardiopulmonary bypass. Pulmonary blood flow is then provided by a systemic–to–pulmonary artery shunt or a bidirectional cavopulmonary connection as appropriate.

This chapter reviews the early and midterm outcome in a subset of neonates with univentricular pathophysiology and aortic obstruction who, in addition, possess the substrate at highest risk for developing subaortic obstruction. These patients were initially managed by off-pump repair of the aortic obstruction plus short-term PAB en route to the ultimate goal of a Fontan procedure.

PATIENTS

From 1984 to 1998, 15 consecutive neonates with single-ventricle hearts and aortic obstruction were seen at the UCLA Medical Center for surgical treatment (Table 1). In 7 patients the anatomy was a single left ventricle, transposed great arteries, with or without atresia or hypoplasia of the left atrioventricular valve (S,L,L). Two infants had unbalanced complete atrioventricular canal defects with left ventricular hypoplasia. All 15 patients had aortic outflow obstruction with or without aortic arch hypoplasia. During this time, other children with univentricular physiology not considered in this analysis were seen at our institution who were postneonatal, without aortic obstruction, or who had previous interventions at other institutions. Neither children with hypoplastic left heart syndrome nor patients in whom PAB or DKS was performed for biventricular repair were included in this study. Nine of 15 patients (60%) had aortic coarctation, whereas the remaining 6 infants (40%) had aortic arch interruption (4 had type A and 2 had type B). The preoperative diagnosis was established by 2-dimensional echocardiography, color flow imaging, and cardiac catheterization. The following variables were evaluated: timing and sequence of surgical interventions and postsurgical outcome. BVF area index measurements were not consistently documented, and unavailability of outdated preoperative echocardio-

TABLE 1.
Summary of Patient Data

Patient	Age (days)	Weight (kg)	Diagnosis	BVF	DKS (mo)	BDG (mo)	Fontan (mo)	Follow-up (mo)	Outcome
1	6	3.8	{S,L,L} L-AV valve atresia, VSD, aortic coarctation	+	3.62	—	—	3.45*	Dead
2	34	2.6	{S,L,L} DILV, TGA, coarctation, aortic arch hypoplasia	+	52.6	—	52.6	164.4	Alive
3	13	4.6	{S,L,L} DILV, TGA, interrupted aortic arch—type A	+	8.7	—	59.3	147.9	Alive
4	14	4.2	{S,L,L} TGA, malaligned VSD, overriding L-AV valve, interrupted aortic arch—type A	+	2.1	—	—	125.3	Alive
5	13	3.3	{S,D,S} DORV, mitral atresia, aortic coarctation, arch hypoplasia	–	—	14.8	46.8	97.6	Alive
6	2	3.5	{S,D,D} TGA, VSD, mitral atresia, overriding tricuspid valve, small RV, interrupted aortic arch—type A	–	—	13.6	13.6	69.1	Alive
7	3	3.3	{S,L,L} L-AV valve atresia, interrupted aortic arch—type B	+	0.8	6.7	—	52.6	Alive
8	7	4.5	{S,D,D} DILV, TGA, VSD, straddling tricuspid valve, small RV, aortic coarctation	–	—	7.0	57.3	74.3	Alive

(continued)

TABLE 1. (continued}

Patient	Age (days)	Weight (kg)	Diagnosis	BVF (mo)	DKS (mo)	BDG (mo)	Fontan (mo)	Follow-up (mo)	Outcome
9	2	2	{S,D,S} mitral stenosis, VSD, interrupted aortic arch—type B	+	3.5	3.5	—	72.1	Alive
10	6	3.0	{S,L,L} DILV, TGA, aortic coarctation, VSD, small RV	+	7.5	—	—	41.8	Alive
11	5	3.4	{S,D,D} DORV, common AV valve, malposed great arteries, VSD, small RV, interrupted aortic arch—type A	—	—	—	—	0.2	Alive
12	4	3	{S,L,L} DILV, TGA, aortic coarctation	+	0.7	11.6	29.9	91.5	Alive
13	6	2.1	{S,D,D} unbalanced AV canal, aortic coarctation	—	—	—	—	33.0	Alive
14	2	3.2	{S,D,S} DORV, crisscross AV valves, straddling tricuspid valve, small RV, aortic coarctation	—	—	26.5	—	29.4	Alive
15	7	3.2	{S,D,S} unbalanced AV canal, small LV, aortic coarctation and arch hypoplasia	—	—	—	—	1.6+	Dead

*This child died 24 hours after DKS operation.
+Late hospital mortality.
Abbreviations: BVF, bulboventricular foramen; *DKS,* Damus-Kaye-Stansel; *BDG,* bidirectional Glenn (bidirectional cavopulmonary anastomosis); *AV,* atrioventricular; *VSD,* ventricular septal defect; *DILV,* double-inlet left ventricle; *TGA,* transposition of the great arteries; *DORV,* double-outlet right ventricle; *RV,* right ventricle; *LV,* left ventricle; (+), important restriction.

grams made a retrospective calculation of geometric dimensions and ventricular septal defect (VSD) area unfeasible.

OPERATIVE MANAGEMENT

All 15 patients underwent simultaneous relief of aortic arch obstruction plus banding of the pulmonary artery trunk via a left lateral thoracotomy. Subclavian flap angioplasty was used for aortic coarctation repair in all cases except one in which a coarctectomy with end-to-end anastomosis was performed. Similarly, subclavian flap angioplasty was used for the neonates with type A interruption of the aortic arch. Two patients underwent left common carotid artery flap augmentation for accompanying arch hypoplasia. Two neonates with interrupted aortic arch were reconstructed with synthetic Gore-tex grafts. This was in the early experience, and both neonates were clinically unstable at the time of repair.

The pulmonary artery bands were tightened to achieve a distal pulmonary artery pressure of 30% to 50% of the systemic blood pressure while maintaining systemic oxygen saturations of 85% to 90% on a fraction of inspired oxygen concentration of 0.50.

The DKS operation was chosen to bypass the subaortic region when the BVF became restrictive. This procedure was performed using single aortic and bicaval cannulation with moderate hypothermia and low-flow cardiopulmonary bypass. Myocardial protection was achieved using antegrade and retrograde intermittent cold-blood cardioplegia. Topical cooling was also used. After arch reconstruction, the myocardium was reperfused using substrate-enriched warm-blood cardioplegia. The main pulmonary artery trunk is transected and anastomosed to a diamond-shaped aortotomy augmented with an autologous glutaraldehyde-treated pericardial patch reinforced with Dacron mesh.[1] Six infants in whom DKS was performed early after PAB had a Gore-tex shunt placed between the innominate-subclavian artery junction to a branch pulmonary artery to supply the pulmonary circulation. Two children well outside the neonatal period during DKS performance had a bidirectional Glenn (BDG) shunt or Fontan procedure at the same operation. Six children have attained the ultimate surgical goal—a Fontan circulation. A modified lateral tunnel Fontan with snare adjustable atrial septal defect was performed. Details of the operative techniques are presented elsewhere.[2]

Patients' clinical charts and operative and diagnostic reports of cardiac catheterization and echocardiograms were reviewed retrospectively. Follow-up was conducted by direct contact with referring physicians or patients and their families. A restrictive BVF was defined by a measurable Doppler gradient from the dominant

ventricle to the aorta or to a VSD that appeared less than half the
size of the aortic annulus.

RESULTS

OUTCOME

The diagnostic patient profiles of the 12 boys and 3 girls are presented in Table 1. The initial surgical intervention was undertak-
en at a median age of 6 days (range, 2-34 days) and median weight
of 3.3 kg (range, 2-4.6 kg). Forty percent (6 of 15) of the infants
arrived at UCLA intubated and acidemic, and required intravenous fluids and sodium bicarbonate. Eighty percent (12 of 15)
required initiation of intravenous prostaglandin and a third (5 of
15) required inotropic agents for perioperative resuscitation. All
main pulmonary arterial trunks were banded after relief of the aortic arch obstruction without cardiopulmonary bypass. Most of the
patients had an imminently restrictive BVF or had subaortic
obstruction after PAB. Eight children (53%) underwent extracardiac bypass of subaortic stenosis by DKS, including a single child
at the time of BDG and Fontan construction, respectively. The
median age at DKS relief of subaortic stenosis was 3.6 months
(range, 0.7-52.6 months). A single patient who did not have
subaortic stenosis pre-Fontan had a BVF obstruction develop after
Fontan operation and is a candidate for future BVF resection.
Seven children (47%) progressed to BDG at a median age of 9.75
months (range, 3.5-26.5 months). Six (40%) of the 15 children
have attained a Fontan circulation at a median age of 49.7 months
(range, 13.6-59.3 months). A single patient did not tolerate the
Fontan circulation at a year of age and was taken down and left
with a BDG and a central shunt. The median number of cardiac
operations that this high-risk group of 15 patients with a univentricular heart and aortic obstruction has undergone is 3 (range, 1-
5; mean, 3.1).

MORTALITY

Two (13.3%) of 15 children (2 per 1,000 person-months of follow-
up; approximate 95% confidence bounds, 0-4.8) have died.

An infant who had a single ventricle of right ventricular (RV)
morphology and a rudimentary left ventricle (LV) giving rise to the
aorta via a VSD, as well as mitral atresia and coarctation, died after
DKS for subaortic stenosis. The immediate postnatal period was
notable for lethargy, cyanosis, and jaundice. The patient had
important hepatic and renal dysfunction and was transferred to
our institution for management. At 6 days of age, after cardiac
catheterization and balloon atrial septostomy, this neonate underwent an initial repair of the coarctation, PAB, and ligation of a

patent ductus arteriosus. Four months later he had systemic out-flow obstruction (40 mm Hg peak systolic gradient), elevated systemic ventricular end-diastolic pressure (15 mm Hg), and a tight PAB (90 mm Hg peak systolic band gradient), and he underwent urgent DKS and a systemic–to–pulmonary artery shunt. The patient had a cardiac arrest in the postoperative period secondary to pulmonary overcirculation from which he was unable to recover despite narrowing the shunt. Postmortem examination was notable for a dilated systemic RV. There was medial hyperplasia of the pulmonary arterioles indicating pulmonary vascular disease and pulmonary congestion. This patient was the first in the series and was not aggressively followed up for early signs of a restrictive BVF.

Another infant with an unbalanced complete atrioventricular (AV) canal (LV hypoplasia), moderate AV valve regurgitation, aortopulmonary window, aortic coarctation, and subaortic stenosis underwent repair of coarctation of the aorta and bilateral branch PAB at 10 days of life. The infant continued to have some respiratory difficulties despite extubation and feeding and 2 weeks later underwent cardiac catheterization to assess AV valve regurgitation. An aortopulmonary window was not confirmed on that study. The intra-atrial and intraventricular communications were unrestrictive. Bilateral branch pulmonary artery bands were tight. There was severe tricuspid regurgitation. The patient returned to the operating room for removal of the branch pulmonary artery bands and placement of a proximal single band about the main pulmonary arterial trunk. The patient was discharged home after a brief episode of sepsis. She died at 2½ months of age after a brief illness at home.

FOLLOW-UP

These children have been followed-up for a median of 69.1 months (range, 0.2-164.4 months).

Three infants (3 per 1,000 person-months of follow-up; approximate 95% confidence bounds, 0-6.4) subsequently had semilunar (pulmonary) valve insufficiency. The severity of pulmonary regurgitation was graded mild after PAB and DKS in all 3 children. Two of the children have undergone a Fontan operation and 1 has undergone a BDG.

An additional 3 children have mild systemic AV valve regurgitation (3 per 1,000 person-months of follow-up; approximate 95% confidence bounds, 0-6.4).

Three infants had recurrent aortic arch gradients after initial repair for aortic interruption (3 per 1,000 person-months follow-up; approximate 95% confidence bounds, 0 to 6.4). Two infants had successful relief of their gradient after balloon angioplasty. One patient was lost to follow-up with an arch gradient of 15 mmHg.

One patient (1 per 1,000 person-months of follow-up; approximate 95% confidence bounds, 0-2.9) had a gradient of 35 mm Hg develop across the DKS anastomosis that was successfully eliminated after balloon angioplasty.

A single patient contracted hepatitis B during the course of a lateral tunnel Fontan procedure, and a year later cardiomyopathy with arrhythmias developed. The patient is being evaluated for possible heart transplantation. One patient had third-degree heart block 6 years after lateral tunnel Fontan and required dual chamber (DDD) pacemaker implantation. The remaining patients are awaiting evaluation for Fontan.

DISCUSSION

The staged Norwood procedure leading to a Fontan circulation was initially designed for the surgical management of hypoplastic left heart syndrome. Although this concept has undergone methodological evolution since its introduction because of intermediate and late attrition, the Fontan circuit has become the therapeutic goal of a host of complex congenital cardiac malformations with a single ventricle as the dominant and common functional theme. Before this trend, the initial results with ventricular septation techniques were unsatisfactory and notable for a high incidence of complete heart block and high mortality.[3,4] Thus, most investigators have largely abandoned these attempts in favor of a circulation without ventricular-arterial coupling of the pulmonary circulation.

Neonates born with a univentricular heart and aortic obstruction pose a particular surgical challenge. The natural history without intervention is dismal, and the surgical strategies that have evolved have been associated with high morbidity and mortality historically.[5] Since these patients with aortic obstruction and single-ventricle physiology usually have a large pulmonary artery and luxuriant flow, early surgical efforts addressed the preservation of the pulmonary vascular bed by constricting the main pulmonary arterial trunk with a band and repairing the aortic obstruction. Several investigators subsequently reported the development of subaortic stenosis that ultimately jeopardized Fontan candidacy.[6-8] This phenomenon was particularly unique to transposition complexes (as in DILV and tricuspid atresia) with a systemic outflow from the dominant ventricle conducted via a VSD (restrictive BVF) and muscular infundibular chamber to the aorta. Other mechanisms of subaortic obstruction caused by a restrictive subaortic conus (DORV) or AV valve tissue (unbalanced A-V canal) are observed in single-ventricle arrangements. The PAB was implicated in the accelerated development of subaortic obstruction secondary to muscular hypertrophy and restriction of the VSD and subaortic area.[6-8] Ventricular hypertrophy, large muscle mass, and reduced compliance have been identified as risk factors for successful Fontan hemodynamics. The work from Norwood and his group has elegantly demonstrated that volume unloading procedures including PAB acutely precipitate geometric changes in the ventricle heralded by smaller cavity and increased wall thickness compromising the systemic pathway.[9] Thus, it is probable that at least these two underlying mechanisms in the univentricular heart —myocardial hypertrophy and volume unloading—are responsible for the emergence of subaortic obstruction after PAB. Other complications associated with a poorly positioned band or migration were reported, including branch pulmonary stenoses, semilunar valve insufficiency, and erosion with aneurysm formation. These observations, noted after long-standing PAB, have threatened this palliative procedure with obscurity. However, recent studies in the current surgical era using PAB for short-term purposes have demonstrated a substantial reduction in morbidity and mortality. Jensen et al.[10] reported their results of initial PAB (with or without aortic arch reconstruction) in 26 infants with DILV or tricuspid atresia and transposed great arteries. A third of the group had associated obstructive arch abnormalities. There were no deaths after PAB with or without arch repair. An important subaortic gradient (defined as a resting gradient between the ascending aorta and LV equal to or greater than 10 mm Hg) developed in more than half (16 of 26) of the patients. Nineteen infants, including an additional 3 without subaortic stenosis, underwent DKS (12 infants) or VSD enlargement (8 infants), alone or with a Glenn (14 infants) or Fontan procedure (15 infants). There were no deaths after 14 Glenn shunts, and 6 (43%) of the patients had simultaneous relief of subaortic obstruction. There were 5 hospital deaths during the study period (mortality rate of 19%). One patient died of ventricular arrhythmias after a DKS, and 4 infants died after Fontan procedure during the hospitalization. Webber et al.,[11] following a similar strategy of short-term PAB and early relief of subaortic stenosis, in 18 consecutive patients with DILV, transposed great arteries, and an obstructive anomaly of the aortic arch (4 had subaortic stenosis), observed 1 death after PAB and arch repair. A single patient with subaortic stenosis died after initial early aortopulmonary bypass. All but 1 of the 16 survivors subsequently had subaortic stenosis, and they underwent a proximal aortopulmonary connection, resulting in 2 early deaths and 1 late death. Twelve of the 13 remaining survivors have attained a Fontan or Glenn repair.

Amin et al.[12] recently demonstrated that the initial PAB for short-term palliation in this subset of patients does not cause important semilunar valvular insufficiency precluding later DKS in patients requiring management of subaortic stenosis. In their retrospective review of 15 patients with single-ventricle physiology and systemic outflow obstruction, no operative mortality was associated with primary PAB or later DKS. Minimal PAB-related complications occurred. Half of their patients attained a Fontan circulation during the study period. These recent reports are consistent with our findings that initial short-term PAB in this population is associated with very low mortality. Aggressive surveillance for detection of subaortic stenosis prompts earlier relief of systemic outflow obstruction and the stimulus for ventricular hypertrophy outside the vulnerable neonatal period, allowing many of these patients to proceed to successful Fontan.

The deleterious effects of irreversible myocardial hypertrophy on Fontan eligibility or attrition has prompted surgical strategies seeking early initial relief of aortic obstruction and the avoidance of PAB. Karl et al.[13] and Lacour-Gayet et al.[14] have advocated a palliative arterial switch operation in newborns with univentricular morphology and subaortic stenosis, trading subaortic for neo-subpulmonary stenosis. This approach has yielded unpredictable pulmonary blood flow requiring a later systemic source (shunt) or banding in the event of too much pulmonary blood flow. The reported numbers of patients undergoing this palliative one-stage arterial switch are low, the follow-up is short, and the ultimate suitability for Fontan operation is undetermined.

A direct attack by muscular resection and enlargement of the BVF or VSD to relief subaortic obstruction has led to instances of postoperative heart block, ventricular dysfunction, and late aneurysm formation—all adverse conditions for optimal Fontan performance.[15] LV apical-to-aortic conduits, designed to bypass the subaortic area, lack long-term durability because of valvular degeneration and distortion with somatic growth of the child.[16]

Damus,[17] Kaye,[18] and Stansel[19] independently described a procedure designed for surgical correction of transposition of the great vessels without coronary transfer that has been applied by many investigators to bypass actual or imminent subaortic obstruction. This extracardiac aortopulmonary bypass procedure requires provision of a reliable source of pulmonary blood flow via systemic–to–pulmonary artery shunt, bidirectional cavopulmonary anastomosis, or total cavopulmonary connection (Fontan) as dictated by the clinical circumstances. Other workers have accomplished this goal with a modified Norwood procedure requiring a period of circulatory arrest.

Brawn et al.[20] reported 9 early deaths in a series of 24 infants with complex forms of single-ventricle physiology and systemic outflow obstruction managed with initial modified Damus plus a 3.5-mm aortopulmonary shunt (early mortality rate of 38%). Ten of the 15 survivors underwent Glenn shunt, with 1 death during the study period (overall mortality rate of 42%).

McElhinney et al.[21] recently reported the outcome of DKS in 21 patients with univentricular physiology and subaortic obstruction, 15 of whom had concomitant arch obstruction. All 17 patients in whom the DKS procedure was performed as a primary palliation had a 3- or 3.5-mm systemic–to–pulmonary artery shunt. Three additional patients beyond the neonatal period underwent concurrent BDG shunt. The early mortality rate was 19%. No late deaths occurred during the study period (median follow-up, 33 months). Nine of the 17 survivors underwent BDG shunt, including 3 attaining a Fontan. An additional patient received a cardiac allograft secondary to cardiomyopathy.

The results for the modified Norwood procedure in this subpopulation of infants without hypoplastic left heart syndrome have improved over time, particularly in centers with high volume and experience.[22,23] Mosca et al.[24] reported a remarkable early mortality of 8% in a group of 38 patients with tricuspid atresia or DILV and ventriculo-arterial discordance undergoing a modified Norwood operation. The majority (92%) of these infants had aortic arch anomalies. There were 5 late deaths (13.1%). Thirty percent and 60% of the surviving patients had undergone a hemi-Fontan and Fontan procedure, respectively.

The initial palliative approach described in this report highlights the low mortality and morbidity of short-term PAB and aortic arch repair without cardiopulmonary bypass in a difficult constellation of neonates born with single-ventricle pathophysiology and obstruction of systemic outflow. It appears that the majority of neonates in this subclassification can undergo PAB regardless of the actual measurement of bulboventricular area index. According to the findings of Matitiau et al.[25] in patients with univentricular physiology and aortic arch obstruction, one would predict an earlier tendency toward subaortic obstruction in our cohort of neonates. They found that the mean initial BVF area index was 1.05 ± 0.6 cm^2/m^2 and was significantly smaller in infants with arch obstruction than in patients without (3.35 ± 1.75 cm^2/m^2) ($P < 0.0001$). These investigators found that all patients with an initial BVF area index of less than 2 cm^2/m^2 who did not undergo early bypass had late obstruction.[25]

Thus, the imminent development of subaortic obstruction is aggressively sought out after PAB and corrected with DKS and a controlled source of pulmonary blood flow. This strategy avoids the potential irreversible effects of chronic PAB on myocardial muscle mass and ventricular compliance, and preserves Fontan eligibility. The spectrum of morphology in infants with functional single ventricle and variable degrees of aortic arch obstruction precludes the recommendation of one surgical strategy over another. Case-by-case application of alternative approaches seems most appropriate based on clinical outcome and institutional experience. The long-term neurodevelopmental effects of circulatory arrest used in the staged Norwood approach or the low-flow cardiopulmonary bypass technique in the DKS strategy in neonates remain unanswered. On the other hand, the low incidence of semilunar valve insufficiency, branch pulmonary stenosis, and mortality indicates that short-term banding of the pulmonary artery is at the very least comparable to the more radical surgical approaches for the univentricular heart designed to avoid the issue of subaortic obstruction. The long-term effects on Fontan eligibility or suitability are not answered by this study but compare to the other strategies in the short-term.

This chapter has focused on results of a single treatment strategy at a single center. In the subpopulation of neonates studied with univentricular hearts, the sample size is small because we reviewed our experience in those children born with aortic arch obstruction and thus, additionally, a high likelihood of having imminent subaortic obstruction. Further limitations include the wide variability in pathologic diagnosis, lack of prospective randomization, and an inability to discern what characteristics might favor one surgical strategy over another.

REFERENCES

1. Gates RN, Laks H, Elami A, et al: Damus-Stansel-Kaye procedure: Current indications and results. *Ann Thorac Surg* 56:111-119, 1993.
2. Laks H, Pearl JM, Haas GS, et al: Partial Fontan: The advantages of an adjustable interatrial communication. *Ann Thorac Surg* 52:1084-1095, 1991.
3. McGoon DC, Danielson GK, Ritter DG, et al: Correction of the univentricular heart with left anterior subaortic outlet chamber. *J Thorac Cardiovasc Surg* 74:218-226, 1977.
4. Stefanelli G, Kirklin JW, Naftel DC, et al: Early and intermediate (10-year) results of surgery for univentricular atrioventricular connection ("single ventricle"). *Am J Cardiol* 54:811, 1984.
5. Moodie DS, Ritter DG, Tajik AJ, et al: Long term follow-up in the unoperated univentricular heart. *Am J Cardiol* 53:1124-1128, 1984.
6. Freedom RM, Sondheimer H, Dische MR, et al: Development of

"subaortic stenosis" after pulmonary artery banding for common ventricle. *Am J Cardiol* 39:78-83, 1977.

7. Freedom RM, Benson LN, Smallhorn JF, et al: Subaortic stenosis, the univentricular heart, and banding of the pulmonary artery: An analysis of the courses of 43 patients with univentricular heart palliated by pulmonary artery banding. *Circulation* 73:758-764, 1986.

8. Franklin RCG, Sullivan ID, Anderson RH, et al: Isolated banding of the pulmonary trunk obsolete for infants with tricuspid atresia and double inlet ventricle with discordant ventriculoarterial connection? Role of aortic arch obstruction and subaortic stenosis. *J Am Coll Cardiol* 1455-1464, 1990.

9. Rychik J, Jacobs ML, Norwood WI: Acute changes in left ventricular geometry after volume reduction surgery. *Ann Thorac Surg* 60:1267-1274, 1995.

10. Jensen RA, Williams RG, Laks H, et al: Usefulness of banding of the pulmonary trunk with single ventricle physiology at risk for subaortic obstruction. *Am J Cardiol* 77:1089-1093, 1996.

11. Webber SA, LeBlanc JG, Keeton BR, et al: Pulmonary artery banding is not contraindicated in double inlet left ventricle with transposition and aortic arch obstruction. *Eur J Cardiothorac Surg* 9:515-520, 1995.

12. Amin Z, Backer CL, Duffy CE, et al: Does banding the pulmonary artery affect pulmonary valve function after the Damus-Kaye-Stansel operation? *Ann Thorac Surg* 66:836-841, 1998.

13. Karl TR, Watterson KG, Sano S, et al: Operations for subaortic stenosis in univentricular hearts. *Ann Thorac Surg* 52:420-428, 1991.

14. Lacour-Gayet F, Serraf A, Fremont L, et al: Early palliation of univentricular hearts with subaortic stenosis and ventriculoarterial discordance. *J Thorac Cardiovasc Surg* 104:1238-1245, 1991.

15. O'Leary PW, Driscoll DJ, Conner AR, et al: Subaortic obstruction in hearts with a univentricular connection to a dominant left ventricle or an anterior subaortic outlet chamber: Results of a staged approach. *J Thorac Cardiovasc Surg* 104:1231-1238, 1992.

16. Frommelt PC, Rocchini AP, Bove EL: Natural history of apical left ventricular to aortic conduits in pediatric patients. *Circulation* 84:213-218, 1991.

17. Damus PS: Letter to the editor. *Ann Thorac Surg* 20:724-725, 1975.

18. Kaye MP: Anatomic correction for transposition of the great arteries. *Mayo Clin Proc* 50:638-640, 1975.

19. Stansel HC Jr: A new operation for d-loop transposition of the great vessels. *Ann Thorac Surg* 19:565-567, 1975.

20. Brawn WJ, Sethia B, Jagtap R, et al: Univentricular heart with systemic outflow obstruction: Palliation by primary Damus procedure. *Ann Thorac Surg* 59:1441-1447, 1995.

21. McElhinney DB, Reddy VM, Silverman NH, et al: Modified Damus-Kaye-Stansel procedure for single ventricle, subaortic stenosis and arch obstruction in neonates and infants: Midterm results and techniques for avoiding circulatory arrest. *J Thorac Cardiovasc Surg* 114:718-726, 1997.

22. Jonas RA, Castenada AR, Lang P: Single ventricle complicated by

subaortic stenosis: Surgical options in infancy. *Ann Thorac Surg* 39:361-366, 1985.

23. Rychik J, Murdison KA, Chin AJ, et al: Surgical management of severe aortic outflow obstruction in lesions other than hypoplastic left heart syndrome: Use of pulmonary artery to aorta anastomosis. *J Am Coll Cardiol* 18:809-816, 1991.
24. Mosca RS, Hennein HA, Kulik TJ, et al: Modified Norwood operation for single left ventricle and ventriculoarterial discordance: An improved surgical technique. *Ann Thorac Surg* 64:1126-1132, 1997.
25. Matitiau A, Geva T, Colan SD, et al: Bulboventricular foramen size in infants with double-inlet left ventricle or tricuspid atresia with transposed great arteries: Influence on initial palliative operation and rate of growth. *J Am Coll Cardiol* 19:142-148, 1992.

CHAPTER 9

Surgical Treatment of Single Ventricle With Aortic Arch Obstruction in Early Life

Christo I. Tchervenkov, M.D., F.R.C.S.C.
Associate Professor of Surgery, McGill University; Director of Cardiovascular Surgery, Montreal Children's Hospital of the McGill University Health Centre, Montreal, Quebec, Canada

John C. Tsang, M.D.
Chief Cardiothoracic Surgery Resident, Montreal Children's Hospital of the McGill University Health Centre, Montreal, Quebec, Canada

R emarkable advances in the surgical treatment of patients with single ventricle have occurred during the past 30 years. The successful application of the Fontan operation has resulted in tremendous optimism for the long-term outcome of these patients. However, the survival in early life is far from ideal, and many patients will never become candidates for the Fontan operation.[1-3] This may be caused by complicating factors resulting from the presence of unfavorable associated lesions or complications of suboptimal initial surgical therapy. Furthermore, despite significant improvement in the early survival after the Fontan operation from continued refinements in surgical technique, improvement in patient selection criteria, and perioperative management, there continues to be a significant attrition of these patients on long-term follow-up.[4,5] Thus, as the next century approaches, one of the remaining challenges in the treatment of patients with congenital heart disease is to optimize the surgical management of the single ventricle physiology. Improvements will require the understanding of not only which factors lead to success, but more importantly the factors that result in failure, so that they can be avoided.

Because of the extreme heterogeneity of this group of patients, the initial surgical approach plays a crucial role in the eventual outcome of the patient and therefore must be tailored to the specific anatomy and associated lesions. This chapter focuses on the challenging combination of single ventricle with aortic arch obstruction (AAO), which has been associated with a very high mortality and whose initial surgical approach has remained highly controversial. The apparent lack of progress primarily has been caused by the relatively small number of such patients seen in each center during a time of rapid evolution and refinement of surgical procedures, and the need for long-term follow-up to decide on the best initial approach.

In this chapter, we review the nomenclature, anatomical aspects, pathophysiology, incidence, natural history, goals of optimal surgical therapy, and current surgical options and outcomes, as well as our experience at the Montreal Children's Hospital. We analyze the overall surgical experience and draw conclusions from the knowledge to date, propose a surgical treatment algorithm, and finally lay out future directions. The specific technical details of the various surgical procedures are not discussed because they are described in detail elsewhere.

NOMENCLATURE

Controversy is ongoing as to what constitutes a single ventricle. A number of other designations have been used, such as common ventricle, double-inlet ventricle, hearts with univentricular atrioventricular connection, or univentricular hearts.[6,7] Furthermore, a number of other pathologic entities have single-ventricle physiology, such as tricuspid atresia, severely unbalanced complete atrioventricular canal, double-outlet right ventricle with left ventricular hypoplasia, and hypoplastic left heart syndrome. Hearts with single-ventricle physiology are therefore an extremely heterogeneous group. In this chapter, we use the term single ventricle predominantly to refer to these kinds of patients. We will focus on the surgical treatment in early life of patients with single ventricle and AAO in an attempt to settle some of the surgical controversies. Although most of the patients considered have hearts with univentricular atrioventricular connection with a main ventricular chamber, a rudimentary chamber supporting the aorta, with a bulboventricular communication between them, excessive pulmonary blood flow, and AAO, other rare variants with single-ventricle physiology are also included in most publications. The classic hypoplastic left heart syndrome, however, will not be part of this discussion.

ANATOMICAL CONSIDERATIONS

In patients with single ventricle, AAO occurs in the absence of pulmonary outflow obstruction. In patients with double-inlet ventricle or tricuspid atresia, AAO is more likely in the presence of ventriculoarterial discordance, with the pulmonary artery arising from the main ventricular chamber and the aorta from the rudimentary outlet ventricular chamber. These two chambers are connected by an interventricular communication otherwise known as the bulboventricular foramen (BVF). In tricuspid atresia, this usually occurs with transposition of the great arteries (TGA), whereas in double-inlet ventricle it may be present when the malposed aorta is supported by a left-sided rudimentary chamber usually of right ventricular morphology. AAO has been hypothesized to develop as a result of diminished aortic flow through a restrictive BVF during development of the great vessels.[8] Matitiau et al.[9] noted that in 16 patients with single ventricle and AAO vs. 12 patients with single ventricle without AAO, there was a significantly smaller BVF index (1.05 ± 0.6 cm^2/m^2 vs. 3.35 ± 1.75 cm^2/m^2). Therefore, even in the absence of a measurable gradient across the systemic outflow tract, the presence of AAO should increase the index of suspicion of potential subaortic stenosis (SAS). Based on these observations, an initial BVF area index of less than 2 cm^2/m^2 has been suggested to be highly predictive of subsequent subaortic obstruction.[9]

The development of SAS in univentricular hearts with discordant ventriculoarterial connections at the BVF can be difficult to assess. The BVF is not perfectly round but rather has a "buttonhole" or elliptical appearance.[10] Therefore, the determination of its size must be made accurately with multiple views such as with 2-dimensional echocardiography rather than from angiography, because even when the largest dimension approaches that of the aorta, the cross-sectional area may be significantly smaller. Franklin et al.[11] observed that patients with an initial BVF-to-aorta ratio of less than 0.8 are at high risk of developing SAS after pulmonary artery banding. Furthermore, Rao[12] noted that there is a natural tendency for the BVF to spontaneously close, again emphasizing the potential for systemic outflow obstruction at this site.

PATHOPHYSIOLOGY

Most patients with single ventricle and AAO are critically ill soon after birth. The absence of pulmonary obstruction leads to pulmonary overcirculation with rapid development of congestive heart failure. In the presence of AAO, the circulation to the lower body is supported by the patent ductus arteriosus. Its closure will result in an acute hypoperfusion of the lower body, precipitating acute renal failure, severe metabolic acidosis, and necrotizing enterocolitis. At the same time, the congestive heart failure will be exacerbated, with acute pulmonary edema and marked cardiomegaly. The rapidly progressing downhill course inevitably is fatal unless the baby is rapidly resuscitated, most importantly with the administration of prostaglandins to reopen the ductus arteriosus, inotropic support of cardiac function, and correction of the acid-base disturbances.

INCIDENCE

The true incidence of AAO associated with single ventricle physiology is difficult to determine because of the extreme heterogeneity of this group of patients. Franklin et al.[11] noted that 30% of patients with double-inlet left ventricle and 20% of patients with tricuspid atresia seen during the first year of life have a single dominant left ventricle, discordant ventriculoarterial connections, and unrestricted pulmonary blood blow. AAO was seen in approximately 50% of these infants.[11] Kirklin[13,14] reported that the incidence of AAO in double-inlet ventricle was 26%, and the incidence in tricuspid atresia was 30%. Castaneda[15] noted that interrupted aortic arch occurs much less frequently, with an incidence of 11% in patients with single ventricle equivalents. A review of data from the Boston's Children's Hospital experience demonstrated that of 162 patients with functional single ventricle, 71 (44%) had excessive pulmonary blood flow. Among this group, 32 patients (45%) had associated AAO.[6]

NATURAL HISTORY

The natural history of this congenital malformation without surgical treatment is overwhelmingly fatal. Franklin et al.[11] noted that of 13 patients with single ventricle, AAO, and without SAS not treated because they were too sick or had too complex anatomy, 12 died in infancy and the remaining child died at 3.5 years. When there was single ventricle, AAO, and SAS at presentation, all 6 patients died in infancy.[11]

The dismal survival of neonates with single ventricle and coarctation of the aorta, despite surgical treatment, is evident in the Congenital Heart Surgeon Society (CHSS) study on the outcome of neonates with coarctation.[16] Among 435 neonates with coarctation from 28 institutions entered in their database during a 2-year period from 1990 to 1992, 32 patients had single ventricle. Only 10 of these patients were alive at the conclusion of this relatively short study period, resulting in a mortality of 69%. This underscores the difficult surgical challenge and that optimal surgical therapy remains an elusive goal. No details are available from the CHSS publication as to the surgical approaches used and their outcomes. The low number of patients despite the large number of centers emphasizes the rarity of this entity.

GOALS OF SURGICAL THERAPY

The goal of initial surgical therapy should be to achieve the highest possible early as well as late survival, while making the patient an ideal candidate for the Fontan operation. Optimal criteria for the Fontan operation are shown in Table 1.[7] Interestingly, the absence of systemic outflow obstruction is not part of the criteria, despite a high mortality rate after the Fontan operation in its presence.[3,5,17] This is implied indirectly under the criteria of normal ventricular function. However, because systemic outflow obstruction, either at the subaortic area or in the aortic arch itself, is so detrimental to the outcome after the Fontan operation, we are proposing that it be included in the criteria outlined in Table 1.

The initial approach to the patient with single ventricle and AAO will be determinant for the ultimate outcome. The establishment of unobstructed systemic circulation is crucial because it will serve to maintain good systolic and diastolic function of the single ventricle. Preservation of competent atrioventricular and

---

TABLE 1.

Optimal Criteria for the Fontan Operation

Normal sinus rhythm

Normal caval and pulmonary venous connections

Normal pulmonary vascular resistance, with a mean pulmonary arterial pressure < 15-20 mm Hg

No significant pulmonary artery branch stenosis that would preclude surgical repair

Pulmonary artery–aortic ratio > 0.75

"Normal" ventricular function

No regurgitation of the systemic atrioventricular valve

Normal diastolic ventricular function

Optimum minimal age: uncertain, but when anatomy and hemodynamics ideal, probably 2-4 years. Until recently, a minimum age of 4 years had been advocated.

Unobstructed systemic circulation (no aortic arch obstruction or subaortic stenosis)*

*This point added by us.

(Modified from Freedom RM: Double-inlet ventricle, in Freedom RM [ed]: *Congenital Heart Diseases: Textbook of Angiocardiography*, vol 2. New York, Futura Publishing, 1997, pp 1201-1260.)

TABLE 2.

Goals of Surgical Treatment of Single Ventricle and AAO

Establishment of unobstructed systemic circulation

Preservation of normal systolic and diastolic function of the single ventricle

Preservation of good function of atrioventricular and semilunar valves

Prevention of pulmonary vascular obstructive disease

Prevention of pulmonary venous obstruction

Prevention of pulmonary artery distortions or stenoses

semilunar valve function will contribute to a good long-term outcome. Of particular importance is the achievement of adequate, but not excessive pulmonary blood flow to prevent the development of pulmonary vascular obstructive disease. The prevention or elimination of pulmonary venous obstruction, particularly in patients with left atrioventricular valve atresia, and the avoidance of pulmonary artery distortions complete the surgical goals (Table 2). The appropriate surgical approach should fulfill these goals and ideally result in the patient becoming an optimal candidate for the Fontan operation, as outlined in Table 1.

SURGICAL OPTIONS AND OUTCOMES

Several surgical approaches have been used over the years for single ventricle with AAO. Although some have been largely abandoned, none has emerged as the clear procedure of choice. Pulmonary artery banding and coarctation repair have been used the longest, whereas the Norwood operation or the palliative arterial switch operation are relatively new additions to the surgical armamentarium. Although the last two options offer renewed optimism, these have also added to the surgical controversy as to what is the best approach. The advantages and disadvantages of the main surgical options currently used are summarized in Table 3. Surgical results with each of these options are presented in Tables 4, 5, and 6.

PULMONARY ARTERY BANDING AND COARCTATION REPAIR

Pulmonary artery banding (PAB) was first described for decreasing pulmonary blood flow and prevention of pulmonary hypertension in 1952 by Muller and Dammann.[18] The combined procedures of PAB and coarctation repair via left thoracotomy have been the traditional approach during infancy to the management of the patient with single ventricle and AAO (Table 4). This has been advocated

TABLE 3.

Surgical Strategies for Single Ventricle With AAO

Primary Procedure	Advantages	Disadvantages
Pulmonary artery band and relief of aortic arch obstruction	Simplicity No need for CPB or DHCA Lower immediate risk	High risk for SAS Need for reoperations for SAS Potential for residual AAO Increased myocardial hypertrophy Pulmonary valve damage precluding DKS Potential for doubly obstructed heart
Proximal pulmonary artery to aortic anastomosis and arch repair (Norwood/DKS)	Avoids potential SAS at BVF and consequent myocardial hypertrophy Bypasses multiple levels of obstruction Greater potential for extensive arch enlargement	Higher risk procedure in neonatal period Shunt physiology Need for CPB or DHCA Distortion of pulmonary valve, PI Potential need for prosthetics in reconstruction
Palliative arterial switch and arch repair	Avoids potential SAS at BVF and consequent myocardial hypertrophy Creation of harmonious aortic root Natural protection of pulmonary bed by BVF	Higher risk procedure in neonatal period Potential for myocardial ischemia from coronary distortion Need for CPB or DHCA Frequent need for shunt to augment pulmonary blood flow Potential for supra-aortic, suprapulmonic obstruction

Abbreviations: DKS, Damus-Kaye-Stansel; *PI,* pulmonary insufficiency.

for the critically ill neonate as a low-risk first-step palliation that does not require cardiopulmonary bypass (CPB) or deep hypothermic circulatory arrest (DHCA). PAB also serves to decrease the volume overload on the single ventricle as well as to protect the pulmonary artery bed from developing pulmonary vascular obstructive disease. However, the use of PAB for single ventricle with dis-

TABLE 4.
Summary of Results of Selected Series on Primary PAB and Relief of AAO

Author	Patients	Results	SAS	Bidirectional Glenn	Fontan	Overall Results
Rothman[52] 1987	10 patients palliated with PAB and CoA repair	No deaths after PAB and CoA repair	All required surgcial relief of SAS; 5 deaths	—	—	Overall early mortality of 50%; uncertain suitability of remaining patients for Fontan
Franklin[11] 1990	33 patients palliated PAB and CoA repair	17 operative and 3 late deaths	13 subsequently had SAS; 4 died awaiting surgery; 5 underwent further palliation with 2 operative deaths	—	4 Fontans with simultaneous repair of SAS; 2 operative deaths; 2 others fulfill Fontan criteria; 1 has PVD	Overall mortality of the group 79%
Huddleston[62] 1993	4 patients palliated with PAB and CoA repair and planned early takedown to a DKS/Glenn or Fontan	No deaths after initial palliation	All patients underwent DKS	3 had Glenn simultaneous with DKS; 1 late death due to arrhythmia	2 had Fontan simultaneous with DKS; 1 early death	Overall mortality of the group 40%

Webber[35] 1995	18 patients	1/1 death after neonatal Norwood; 17 PAB and CoA repair; 1 death	15/16 remaining patients subsequently had SAS at a median of approximately 8 months (DKS/APW)	1 takedown of Fontan to Glenn for intractable effusions 4 Glenn's performed with SAS relief	7 successful Fontans 1 patient unaccounted	Overall mortality 28%; 2 operative deaths after SAS relief and 1 late death
Jensen[36] 1996	8 patients palliated with PAB and CoA repair	No deaths after PAB and CoA repair	All subsequently had SAS requiring DKS at a median of ~11 months	1/6	5/6	Overall mortality 25%; 2 deaths; 1 death after DKS; 1 death after Fontan and VSD enlargement
Amin[31] 1998	5 patients palliated with PAB and CoA repair	No deaths after PAB and CoA repair	All subsequently had DKS	4	5/5	Overall mortality 0%
Tchervenkov 1987-1996	5 PAB and arch repair	3 deaths	2; 1 BVF enlargement	2	1	Overall mortality 60%

Abbreviations: CoA, coarctation; PVD, pulmonary vascular disease; DKS, Damus-Kaye-Stansel; APW, aortopulmonary window; VSD, ventricular septal defect.

TABLE 5.
Summary of Results of Selected Series on Primary Norwood/DKS

Author	Patients	Results	SAS	Bidirectional Glenn	Fontan	Overall Results
Matitiau[9] 1992	12 patients treated with DKS	3 early deaths and 2 late deaths	None	2 Glenn procedures	5 Fontans	Overall mortality 42%
Brawn[43] 1995	14 patients treated with primary DKS	2 early deaths	None	9 Glenn procedures; 3 patients unaccounted	—	Overall mortality 14%
Kanter[41] 1995	6 patients treated with primary Norwood	One operative death	None	5 Glenn	All 5 deemed to be suitable Fontan candidates	Overall mortality 17%
Jacobs[40] 1995	18 patients treated with primary Norwood	5 deaths	None	—	All 13 deemed to be suitable Fontan candidates	Overall mortality 28%

Mosca[42] 1997	35 patients treated with primary Norwood	3 early and 5 late deaths	None	9 Hemi-Fontan procedures	18 successful Fontans	Overall mortality 23%
McElhinney[46] 1997	10 patients treated with primary DKS	1 early death	None	8 Glenn	1 Fontan	Overall mortality 10%
Tchervenkov 1987-1991	5 patients treated with primary Norwood	4 early deaths	None	—	1 Fontan	Overall mortality 80%
Tchervenkov 1995-1999	5 patients treated with primary Norwood	No early deaths	None	3 Glenn	1 Fontan; 2 deemed to be suitable Fontan candidates	Overall mortality 0%

Abbreviation: DKS, Damus-Kaye-Stansel.

TABLE 6.
Summary of Results of Palliative Arterial Switch

Author	Patients	Results	SAS	Bidirectional Glenn	Fontan	Overall Results
Karl[48] 1991	5 patients treated with primary palliatve arterial switch	1 operative death and 1 late death	None	—	1 Fontan; 2 awaiting Fontan	Overall mortality 40%
Lacour-Gayet[49] 1992	5/7 patients treated with palliative switch; 2/7 patients treated with PAB and CoA repair followed by palliative switch	2 early deaths	None	—	5 alive and well awaiting Fontan	Overall mortality 29%

Abbreviation: CoA, coarctation.

cordant ventriculoarterial connection physiology has decreased since the report by Freedom et al.,[19] who noted an 84.4% (27 of 32 patients) incidence of SAS in those patients treated initially with PAB. This report does not, however, comment on whether the patients had known AAO. Subsequently, others have described similar development of subaortic obstruction after PAB, which is known to be a risk factor for mortality after the Fontan operation.[20,21] More strikingly, Franklin et al.[11] reported in a retrospective study that of 33 patients with single left ventricle, discordant ventriculoarterial connection, and AAO treated with PAB and aortic arch repair, only 5 patients survived until the end of the follow-up period. Among this group, only 2 have successfully undergone the Fontan operation, 2 others fulfill the Fontan criteria, and 1 patient has pulmonary vascular obstructive disease. All the patients in this series had SAS by 3 years of age.

The presence of preexisting BVF obstruction in the neonate with single ventricle and AAO has generally been considered a contraindication to PAB. However, in the setting of a critically ill neonate in congestive heart failure, with a large patent ductus, it may be difficult to assess the pressure gradient across the foramen, even when provoked with isoproterenol. The associated AAO further diminishes any potentially detectable gradients. Coarctation or AAO should in itself suggest the presence of obstruction to systemic flow at the BVF as suggested by Matitiau et al.[9] Therefore, SAS should be anticipated in the setting of a single ventricle with AAO because of the morphological substrate inherent to these defects. Donofrio et al.[22] suggested that the volume unloading of the ventricle caused by PAB may further alter ventricular geometry, resulting in an acute diminution of BVF size and worsening the SAS. The placement of a PAB in the setting of SAS results in the creation of a doubly obstructed heart, accelerating the process of myocardial hypertrophy, ischemia and fibrosis, and eventual myocardial failure. Freedom et al.[19] further emphasized that when SAS develops after PAB, the ventricular hypertension leads to elevation of distal pulmonary artery pressures despite the PAB, leaving an unprotected pulmonary vascular bed. This is caused by the myocardial hypertrophy altering ventricular compliance and impairing atrial emptying.

The development of SAS after PAB requires further reintervention. This has included the creation of a proximal pulmonary artery–to–aorta anastomoses, which some groups have advocated as the primary procedure in neonates with single ventricle and AAO. Other reported techniques for relieving SAS after PAB include creation of an aorto-pulmonary window proximal to the PAB.[23] However, this technique reportedly has been associated with the development of aortic insufficiency and aneurysms of the sinus of Valsalva.[23] Another technique is the creation of a conduit between the pulmonary trunk proximal to the PAB and the descending aorta.[7] Alternative options for the surgical relief of SAS after PAB include enlargement of BVF either via ventriculotomy or aortotomy. This has been used successfully in several reports.[24,25] Concerns with this approach involve potential damage to the atrioventricular node despite an improved knowledge of the region.[26] Furthermore, the stenosis can potentially occur at the annular level, resulting in incomplete relief of the SAS.[27] Other possible complications with this approach include coronary injury and development of aneurysms at the systemic ventriculotomy site. Another concern for direct enlargement of the BVF is the potential malattachment of atrioventricular valve tissue about the margins of the defect, which may make the resection impossible or damage valve function subsequently.[28] The technique of apical ventricular to descending aorta conduit for the relief of SAS rarely has been used in recent years.[29]

PAB also can lead to damage to the pulmonary valve, with resultant pulmonary insufficiency caused by proximal placement of the band[25] or development of branch pulmonary artery stenoses secondary to distal migration.[19] It has also been reported that the pulmonary insufficiency from severe valve damage after proximal placement of the PAB may be echographically undetectable.[30] However, several studies suggest that meticulous placement of the PAB should avoid the development of such complications.[31,32]

Another potential drawback of PAB and aortic arch repair may be incomplete relief of the AAO when approached via a left thoracotomy.[33] These patients often have a tubular hypoplasia of the aortic arch up to the level of the coarctation. In the largest single institution series on neonatal coarctation for Marie-Lannelongue in Paris, tubular hypoplasia of the aortic arch was present in 93% of patients with complex intracardiac lesions.[34] These authors also observed that complete or complex aortic arch hypoplasia was more prevalent in that group of patients. Techniques such as subclavian flap angioplasty or coarctectomy and even extended end-to-end anastomosis may not be able to adequately address the hypoplasia of the arch. Interruption of the aortic arch may also be difficult to repair via a left thoracotomy, requiring the use of a prosthetic tube graft with no growth potential. Residual AAO would further increase the afterload on the heart, increase pulmonary blood flow, and accelerate the process of myocardial hypertrophy.[15]

The proponents of PAB have suggested that the poor outcome and increased risk of development of SAS with this approach reported by others is caused by the excessively long duration of

PAB.[35,36] Some of these groups advocate relief of AAO and PAB in the neonatal period as long as there is no preexisting severe SAS.[35] Subsequently, there should be a rigorous surveillance by echocardiography for the development of SAS. The majority of these patients ultimately did have SAS within the first year and were usually treated quickly after detection with a variety of procedures often coupled with a superior cavo-pulmonary anastomosis as an intermediate-stage procedure before the Fontan operation.[35,36] Webber et al.[35] described 18 patients with double-inlet left ventricle, TGA, and AAO. One patient underwent a neonatal Norwood procedure and died. The remaining 17 patients underwent aortic arch repair and PAB with 1 early death. Among the survivors, 15 of 16 patients required relief of SAS with 3 subsequent deaths. Twelve of the 13 patients have undergone the Fontan operation or a bidirectional cavopulmonary anastomosis along with persistent relief of SAS. Amin et al.[31] reported no mortality in 5 patients treated with primary PAB and coarctation repair followed by early Damus-Kaye-Stansel (DKS) procedure. All ultimately had completion of their palliation with the Fontan operation. Jensen et al.[36] described 26 patients at University of California at Los Angeles (UCLA) with single-ventricle physiology. In this cohort, 8 patients had associated AAO and underwent PAB and aortic arch repair. All of these patients subsequently had SAS that was relieved by an early DKS, with 1 death. A second patient died after a Fontan operation and had a very high subaortic gradient preoperatively. The other 6 patients have successfully progressed to a Fontan operation or a cavopulmonary anastomosis. However, 4 of these 6 remaining patients have significant residual subaortic gradients, potentially affecting their long-term outcome. An update of this UCLA experience was presented by Odim et al.[37] at the 1999 meeting of the Society of Thoracic Surgeons. Of 15 neonates with single ventricle and AAO undergoing PAB and relief of AAO as primary palliation, 13 were alive at the end of the follow-up period.[37] Seven infants have required a DKS procedure for subaortic obstruction at a median age of 4 months. Seven patients have undergone bidirectional cavopulmonary anastomoses, whereas 6 have had the Fontan procedure with one takedown to a Glenn. Two of the patients have been deemed not suitable for a Fontan operation. Although these recent results certainly create optimism with this approach, SAS remains a significant problem requiring long-term follow-up before definitive conclusions.

NORWOOD AND DAMUS-KAYE-STANSEL OPERATIONS

The application of the Norwood principle to patients with single ventricle complicated by SAS was first theoretically eluded to by

Penkoske et al.[23] in 1984 as a means of surgical palliation. In 1985, Jonas et al.[8] applied the Norwood principle as a secondary procedure. They had observed in three patients the rapid development of severe SAS after the application of a PAB. The first two patients had also undergone repair of interrupted aortic arch with a Gore-Tex tube graft and coarctation of the aorta by subclavian flap aortoplasty, respectively. The third patient had a normal aortic arch. All three successfully underwent a modified DKS, closure of the distal main pulmonary artery, and a systemic pulmonary shunt at 4, 9, and 10 weeks of age. None of these patients had proceeded to the Fontan operation in the short follow-up reported. In 1990, we reported the successful use of a primary Norwood operation in a neonate with tricuspid atresia, transposition, restrictive BVF, and AAO. Since then, this patient has successfully undergone the Fontan operation.[38]

The construction of a proximal pulmonary artery–to–aorta anastomosis of the Norwood variety or DKS type with a concomitant systemic-pulmonary shunt has been advocated by several groups as the primary procedure for the neonate with single ventricle and AAO (Table 5). This early aggressive approach is able to bypass multiple levels of obstruction at the same time. Because the proximal main pulmonary artery is used as an egress into the systemic circulation, the presence or development of SAS becomes irrelevant. This option also may reduce the need for multiple reoperations to deal with the SAS secondary to PAB. The main drawback with this approach has been the increased risk of a complex operation during the neonatal period requiring CPB and DHCA. The unstable postoperative hemodynamics requiring a perfect balance between the systemic and pulmonary circulations in the presence of a shunt physiology further complicates the postoperative management. Rychik et al.[39] reported on the use of the Norwood operation for lesions other than hypoplastic left heart syndrome in 1991. Within a subgroup of their patients with single ventricle and AAO, the survival to 18 months was 54%. Subsequent reports and modifications of techniques have yielded more favorable results. Jacobs et al.[40] in an update of the Philadelphia experience with the Norwood operation for lesions other than hypoplastic left heart syndrome had an overall mortality of 28%, with the 13 of 18 survivors all deemed to be good Fontan candidates. In a smaller series from Kanter et al.,[41] 5 of 6 patients successfully underwent the Norwood procedure as a first-stage palliation. All survivors also were reported to be good candidates for the Fontan procedure. Mosca et al.[42] described a series of 35 patients with single ventricle and AAO treated with a primary Norwood procedure. They reported 3 early deaths and 5 late deaths. All survivors were evaluated as being suitable candidates for or have undergone the Fontan operation. They noted the BVF size preoperatively and postoperatively. Interestingly, although the absolute size of the restrictive BVF did increase in 50% of the patients, when this was indexed to body surface area, there was an overall decrease in size.

Ilbawi et al.[27] also have been advocates of a primary pulmonary-to-systemic anastomosis in single ventricle equivalents with AAO because they noted that severe SAS consistently developed in these patients. Their technique involves an interposition of a Gore-tex tube graft between the pulmonary artery and the aortic arch to descending aorta that is opened from the hypoplastic arch to the coarctation. They noted that their patients with single ventricle and SAS (with or without AAO) had significantly lower ventricular muscle mass and mass-to-volume ratios when they were treated with primary pulmonary artery–aortic anastomosis vs. PAB followed by subsequent relief of SAS. Furthermore, the former group had good outcomes after the Fontan operation, whereas the group palliated first with PAB and coarctation repair had a high perioperative mortality and required takedown of the Fontan because of low cardiac output and high venous pressures.

The DKS principle has been applied as a primary procedure to palliate single ventricle with AAO as well as SAS by several other groups (Table 5). Brawn et al.[43] modified this procedure to allow for arch enlargement by the pulmonary artery trunk. They had 2 of 14 such patients die early. Subsequent studies have revealed the remaining patients to be good candidates for the Fontan operation. One of the concerns of early DKS connection is the potential development of pulmonary insufficiency, which may adversely affect the outcome of the eventual Fontan operation.[44] This occurred more frequently when it was performed as a direct proximal pulmonary artery end-to-side anastomosis to the ascending aorta. McElhinney et al.[45] have applied a modified DKS technique first described by Laks et al.[46] to avoid distortion of the semilunar valves and allow for reconstruction without the use of exogenous materials. In a subgroup of 10 patients with single ventricle and AAO, there was 1 death. The 9 survivors have undergone either a bidirectional cavopulmonary anastomosis or an extracardiac Fontan operation.

All of these techniques, although carrying different names and technical variations, have the same overall principles of using the main pulmonary artery as an additional egress from the heart into the systemic circulation and a shunt physiology postoperatively.

PALLIATIVE ARTERIAL SWITCH OPERATION

Another proposed alternative for patients with single ventricle, AAO, and increased pulmonary blood flow is a palliative arterial switch operation (ASO; Table 6). This was described by Freedom et al.[47] in 1980 for the palliation of an older child with tricuspid atresia and TGA with SAS after PAB in combination with Fontan operation. The premise of this approach is that in the presence of AAO, there is a very high likelihood for the development of SAS. The performance of a palliative ASO transfers the subaortic obstruction to the subpulmonary level, at the same time creating a natural limitation of pulmonary blood flow. The protection of the pulmonary vasculature by the restrictive BVF after the ASO potentially avoids the difficulties of a shunt-dependent physiology. However, the restriction of pulmonary blood flow by the BVF may be greater than expected because the unobstructed left ventricular outflow tract preferentially promotes flow through the aorta. Thus, the pulmonary blood flow is unpredictable, and there is a potential need for a subsequent systemic-to-pulmonary shunt should the BVF decrease in size over time. The ASO is also felt to allow for the reconstruction of a harmonious aortic root without the use of prosthetic materials as the large pulmonary artery is pulled up toward the distal aortic anastomosis. Improvement in the techniques of ASO has resulted in safer coronary artery transfers. Although an easier Fontan anastomosis is anticipated because of the anterior translocation of the pulmonary artery, there is also a potential for supravalvar pulmonary stenosis after the ASO.

Experience with the palliative ASO has been limited, and the suitability for the Fontan operation has not been clearly detailed in the reported series. Karl et al.[48] presented their experience in 1991 with SAS in univentricular hearts. Within their report, there were five neonates with single ventricle (either tricuspid atresia or double-inlet left ventricle), TGA, and AAO. These newborns had SAS diagnosed and underwent the ASO, atrial septectomy, and aortic arch repair. There was one operative death caused by neoaortic valve incompetence and one late death at 3½ months felt to be related to probable recoarctation. One of the three survivors had undergone a Fontan procedure and was reported to be in New York Heart Association (NYHA) Class I. The other two patients both required subsequent modified Blalock-Taussig shunts but were reported to be well and awaiting Fontan procedures.

Lacour-Gayet et al.[49] have also reported their experience with palliative ASO for single ventricle. In their series of seven patients with single ventricle equivalents and AAO, two patients underwent primary palliation with PAB and coarctation repair and subsequently required palliative ASO because of the development of

SAS. The other five patients underwent a palliative ASO as their primary operation. The transfer of the SAS to subpulmonic stenosis required placement of a systemic-pulmonary shunt in six of the seven patients either during or after the ASO. There was one operative death felt to be related to coronary compression and one late death at 6 months suspected to be related to myocardial ischemia. Four of the survivors are awaiting Fontan operations, whereas the fifth patient had satisfactory right ventricular growth (patient with TGA, VSD, and hypoplastic right ventricle).

ALTERNATIVE SURGICAL APPROACHES

Simultaneous PAB, coarctation repair, and enlargement of the BVF rarely has been used in the neonatal period. Serraf et al.[50] felt that this approach should be limited to the older child because the exposure of the subaortic area can be difficult and the addition of the PAB can result in recurrence of the stenosis.

Another uncommonly used therapy is the apical left ventricular aortic conduit. This surgical option has been used to treat older infants who have subsequently developed SAS.[11] Its use in the neonatal period may be limited by the subsequent need to change the synthetic valved conduit because of degeneration and dysfunction as well as potential damage to ventricular function.[51] In 1984, Penkoske[23] described the use of an apico-aortic conduit with coarctation repair and PAB in a neonate, with the patient dying intraoperatively. Among their series of patients, Rothman et al.[52] described two infants with AAO and single ventricle who were treated with apico-aortic conduits after PAB and coarctation repair. Both infants subsequently died.

Orthotopic heart transplantation has been used as a form of therapy in those patients with very poor function of the single ventricle precluding any type of palliative approach.[50] Results would be expected to be similar to the survival of those neonates undergoing heart transplantation for hypoplastic left heart syndrome.[53]

EXPERIENCE AT THE MONTREAL CHILDREN'S HOSPITAL

At our institution, we have dealt with 15 patients with single ventricle and AAO from 1987 to 1999. During the early experience, both the Norwood approach and PAB and aortic arch repair were used; however, since 1990 we have not used the latter approach.

Five patients were treated with primary PAB and aortic arch repair (Table 4). There was one early death and two late deaths. Two of the patients had received their PAB and arch repair at another institution and were referred for further treatment. Both required subsequent reintervention for recurrent arch obstruction with concomitant Glenn procedure. One child had severe SAS requiring a DKS. However, at the time of operation, the pulmonary valve was nonexistent, damaged by what appeared to be a proximal placement of the PAB. Therefore, the BVF was enlarged causing complete heart block. This patient has since successfully undergone the Fontan operation. The other patient had the substrate for SAS after the PAB and was to undergo a DKS with the revision of arch repair and Glenn procedure. However, on opening the pulmonary artery, there were several perforations in the central portions of the pulmonary valve leaflets precluding its use in a DKS procedure. This patient underwent successful aortic arch repair revision with a Glenn procedure, and the status of the SAS is being followed. These two patients, despite successful palliation to date, again illustrate some of the pitfalls associated with PAB.

Of the early experience from 1987 to 1991 with the Norwood strategy, one of five patients survived and has had a successful Fontan (Table 5). However, since 1995, five other neonates with single ventricle and AAO have been treated with primary Norwood operation and all have survived. Three of the five subsequently had an intermediate Glenn procedure. Two of these patients have progressed to a successful Fontan operation, whereas the other one is a good candidate and will have the Fontan operation in the summer. The remaining two patients are alive and well, awaiting the Glenn operation (Table 5). Therefore, our recent experience with the Norwood operation for these patients is very encouraging, and we feel that it will ultimately emerge as the procedure of choice for the patient with single ventricle and AAO.

ANALYSIS OF SURGICAL EXPERIENCE

The optimal surgical approach to the patient with single ventricle and AAO remains controversial. It is difficult to compare the various surgical options because of the small numbers of patients in each series, which often represent only a subset of a larger group of patients discussed. The patient series are also collected over an extended period during which there has been evolution in surgical techniques and experience. As well, the specialization of a center in one technique or approach results in a surgical expertise that is often not reproducible in all centers. Furthermore, although the surgical options may be similar in principle, there are multiple technical variations that are applied by each center. Finally, outcomes of each approach are not clearly defined because the patients are at varying stages of palliation toward the ultimate Fontan operation, and suitability for the Fontan operation is not always equally determined.

The ultimate goal in the treatment of these patients remains the best possible survival coupled with optimization for the Fontan operation. This requires a protected pulmonary vascular bed, well-developed and undistorted pulmonary arteries, an unobstructed pulmonary venous pathway, and good function of the atrioventricular and semilunar valves. However, the factors that repeatedly have been shown to be critical in the success of the Fontan operation are good systolic and diastolic function of the single systemic ventricle and prevention of abnormal myocardial hypertrophy.[17,54-56] The anatomical substrate of the patient with single ventricle and AAO has a strong propensity toward the development of subaortic obstruction at the BVF. When SAS is left unrecognized and for prolonged periods, the result is myocardial hypertrophy with a stiff and fibrotic systemic ventricle that can ultimately result in a failed Fontan operation.[10] The additional afterload of incomplete relief of AAO will further compromise the integrity of the systemic ventricle. Criteria for the BVF that is at high risk for development of SAS have generally been suggested to be a BVF-to-aortic ratio of less than 0.8[11] or a BVF index of 2 cm^2/m^2.[9] Therefore, the early recognition and elimination of subaortic obstruction is critical in the ultimate palliation of the patient with single ventricle and AAO.

The traditional approach of PAB and aortic arch repair followed by the Fontan operation at an older age has been shown by both Freedom et al.[19] and Franklin et al.[11] to result in dismal outcomes with high mortality. The inevitable progression of SAS and its concomitant adverse effects requiring multiple major reoperations have led many centers to implement other strategies to deal with this complex congenital anomaly. The application of a primary, direct proximal pulmonary artery–to–ascending aorta anastomosis by either a Norwood or modified DKS techniques despite early concerns of high mortality and dependence on a shunt physiology has led recently to promising results in the palliation of these patients. This allows for a bypass of the restrictive BVF while allowing for repair of aortic obstruction in a more uniform manner. The additional staging to the Fontan with Hemi-Fontan[57,58] or bidirectional cavo-pulmonary anastomosis[59,60] has made this an attractive alternative to the traditional approach. The innovative use of the more technically challenging approach of palliative ASO with aortic arch repair may also have a sound physiologic basis. However, this approach has yet to prove that it can consistently lead to suitable and optimal Fontan candidates, and its results may not be reproducible across many centers. The recent renewed interest in the use of initial PAB and relief of AAO followed by vigorous surveillance for SAS and early intervention,

PROPOSED ALGORITHM OF TREATMENT FOR PATIENTS WITH SINGLE VENTRICLE AND AORTIC ARCH OBSTRUCTION

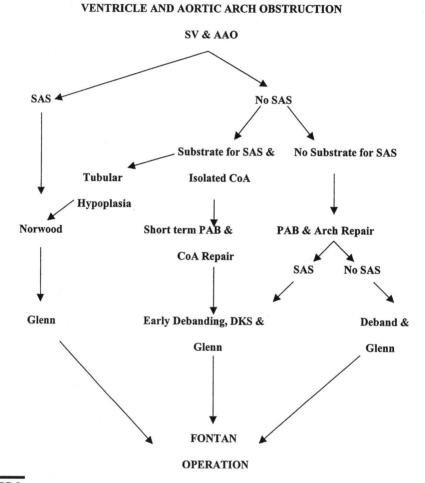

FIGURE 1.
Proposed algorithm for treatment of patients with single ventricle *(SV)* and aortic arch obstruction *(AAO)*. Abbreviation: CoA, coarctation.

coupled with the use of an intervening staging operation, may call for reevaluation of this "dinosaur."[61]

Based on our own experience and that of the others summarized in this chapter, we are proposing an algorithm for the management of the patient with single ventricle and AAO (Fig 1).

FUTURE DIRECTIONS

As with most questions in congenital cardiac surgery, because of the limited numbers of patients and wide distribution of clinical centers that treat these infants, it is impossible to definitively address the optimal treatment strategy in a randomized prospective trial. Furthermore, different centers develop specific expertise because of the implementation of institutional policies toward one approach versus another. However, the only means to attempt to resolve the issue of the optimal approach to the patient with single ventricle and AAO will be through multi-institutional prospective follow-up. By defining criteria so as to attain a more homogenous population and establishing the measures of follow-up as well as standard parameters for assessing Fontan candidacy, this may allow over time the generation of a large enough database to address this complicated issue. Ultimately, by understanding the pathophysiology and morphological substrate of this group of patients and by applying the surgical strategy best suited for each patient, the optimal outcome hopefully will be achieved.

DEDICATION

I dedicate this chapter to my father, Dr. Ivan C. Tchervenkov, who unexpectedly passed away during its preparation. His unparalleled commitment to education, hard work, and family, as well as his unconditional dedication to his patients, will never be forgotten. He will forever remain a guiding light.

—Christo I. Tchervenkov, M.D.

REFERENCES

1. Dick M, Fyler DC, Nadas AS: Tricuspid atresia: Clinical course in 101 patients. *Am J Cardiol* 36:327-337, 1975.
2. Tam CKH, Lightfoot NE, Finlay CD, et al: Course of tricuspid atresia in the Fontan era. *Am J Cardiol* 63:589-593, 1989.
3. Franklin RC, Spiegelhalter DJ, Sullivan ID, et al: Tricuspid atresia presenting in infancy: Survival and suitability for the Fontan operation. *Circulation* 87:427S-439S, 1993.
4. Cohen AJ, Cleveland DG, Dyck J, et al: Results of the Fontan procedure for patients with univentricular heart. *Ann Thorac Surg* 52:1266-1271, 1991.
5. Fontan F, Kirklin J, Fernandez G, et al: Outcome after a "perfect" Fontan operation. *Circulation* 81:1520-1536, 1990.
6. Castaneda AR, Jonas RA, Mayer JE Jr, et al: Single-ventricle tricuspid atresia, in Castaneda AR, Jonas RA, Mayer JE Jr, et al (eds): *Cardiac Surgery of the Neonate and Infant.* Philadelphia, WB Saunders, 1994, pp 249-272.
7. Freedom RM: Double-inlet ventricle, in Freedom RM (ed): *Congenital Heart Diseases: Textbook of Angiocardiography,* vol 2. New York, Futura Publishing, 1997, pp 1201-1260.
8. Jonas RA, Castaneda AR, Lang P: Single ventricle (single- or double-inlet) complicated by subaortic stenosis: Surgical options in infancy. *Ann Thorac Surg* 39: 361S-366S, 1985.

9. Matitiau A, Geva T, Colan SD, et al: Bulboventricular foramen size in infants with double-inlet left ventricle or tricuspid atresia with transposed great arteries: Influence on initial palliative operation and rate of growth. *J Am Coll Cardiol* 19:142S-148S, 1992.

10. Freedom RM: Subaortic obstruction and the Fontan operation. *Ann Thorac Surg* 66:649S-652S, 1998.

11. Franklin RC, Sullivan ID, Anderson RH, et al: Is banding of the pulmonary trunk obsolete for infants with tricuspid atresia and double inlet ventricle with a discordant ventriculoarterial connection? Role of aortic arch obstruction and subaortic stenosis [see comments]. *J Am Coll Cardiol* 16:1455-1464, 1990.

12. Rao PS: Subaortic obstruction after pulmonary artery banding in patients with tricuspid atresia and double-inlet left ventricle and ventriculoarterial discordance (letter). *J Am Coll Cardiol* 18:1585S-1586S, 1991.

13. Kirklin JW, Barratt-Boyce BG: Double inlet ventricle and atretic atrioventricular valve, in Kirklin JW, Barratt-Boyce BG (eds): *Cardiac Surgery*, vol 2. New York, Churchill Livingstone, 1998, pp 1549-1580.

14. Kirklin JW, Barratt-Boyce BG: Tricuspid atresia and the Fontan operation, in Kirklin JW, Barratt-Boyce BG (eds): *Cardiac Surgery*, vol 2. New York, Churchill Livingstone, 1993, pp 1055-1104.

15. Castaneda AR, Jonas RA, Mayer JE Jr, et al: Interrupted aortic arch, in Castaneda AR, Jonas RA, Mayer JE Jr, et al (eds): *Cardiac Surgery of the Neonate and Infant*. Philadelphia, WB Saunders, 1994, pp 353-362.

16. Quaegubeur JM, Jonas RM, Weinberg AD, et al: Outcomes in seriously ill neonates with coarctation of the aorta. *J Thorac Cardiovasc Surg* 108:841-854, 1994.

17. Kirklin JK, Blackstone EH, Kirklin JW, et al: The Fontan operation: Ventricular hypertrophy, age, and date of operation as risk factors. *J Thorac Cardiovasc Surg* 92:1049-1064, 1986.

18. Muller WHJ, Dammann FJJ: The treatment of certain congenital malformations of the heart by the creation of pulmonic stenosis to reduce pulmonary hypertension and excessive pulmonary blood flow: A preliminary report. *Surg Gynecol Obstet* 95:213-219, 1952.

19. Freedom RM, Benson LN, Smallhorn JF, et al: Subaortic stenosis, the univentricular heart, and banding of the pulmonary artery: An analysis of the courses of 43 patients with univentricular heart palliated by pulmonary artery banding. *Circulation* 73:758S-764S, 1986.

20. Coles JG, Kielmanowicz S, Freedom RM, et al: Surgical experience with the modified Fontan procedure. *Circulation* 76:61S-66S, 1987.

21. DeLeon SY, Ilbawi MN, Idriss FS, et al: Fontan type operation for complex lesions. Surgical considerations to improve survival. *J Thorac Cardiovasc Surg* 92:1029S-1037S, 1986.

22. Donofrio MT, Jacobs ML, Norwood WI, et al: Early changes in ventricular septal defect size and ventricular geometry in the single left ventricle after volume-unloading surgery. *J Am Coll Cardiol* 26:1008S-1015S, 1995.

23. Penkoske PA, Freedom RM, Williams WG, et al: Surgical palliation of subaortic stenosis in the univentricular heart. *J Thorac Cardiovasc Surg* 87:767S-781S, 1984.

24. Newfeld EA, Nikaidoh H: Surgical management of subaortic stenosis in patients with single ventricle and transposition of the great vessels. *Circulation* 76:29S-33S, 1987.

25. Cheung HC, Lincoln C, Anderson RH, et al: Options for surgical repair in hearts with univentricular atrioventricular connection and subaortic stenosis. *J Thorac Cardiovasc Surg* 100:672S-681S, 1990.

26. Anderson RH, Ho SY: The pathology of subaortic obstruction. *Ann Thorac Surg* 66:644S-648S, 1998.

27. Ilbawi MN, DeLeon SY, Wilson WR, et al: Advantages of early relief of subaortic stenosis in single ventricle equivalents. *Ann Thorac Surg* 52:842-849, 1991.

28. Freedom RM, Trusler GA: Arterial switch for palliation of subaortic stenosis in single ventricle and transposition: No mean feat (editorial)! *Ann Thorac Surg* 52:415S-416S, 1991.

29. Norwood WI, Lang P, Castaneda AR, et al: Management of infants with left ventricular outflow obstruction by conduit interposition between the ventricular apex and thoracic aorta. *J Thorac Cardiovasc Surg* 68:771, 1983.

30. Tchervenkov CI: Discussion of Amin Z, Backer CL, Duffy CE, et al: Does banding the pulmonary artery affect pulmonary valve function after the Damus-Kaye-Stansel operation? *Ann Thorac Surg* 66:836-841, 1998.

31. Amin Z, Backer CL, Duffy CE, et al: Does banding the pulmonary artery affect pulmonary valve function after the Damus-Kaye-Stansel operation? *Ann Thorac Surg* 66:836-841, 1998.

32. Horowitz MD, Culpepper WS, Williams LC, et al: Pulmonary artery banding: Analysis of a 25 year experience. *Ann Thorac Surg* 48:444-450, 1989.

33. Castaneda AR, Jonas RA, Mayer JE Jr, et al: Aortic coarctation, in Castaneda AR, Jonas RA, Mayer JE Jr, et al (eds): *Cardiac Surgery of the Neonate and Infant.* Philadelphia, WB Saunders, 1994, p 342.

34. Conte S, Lacour-Gayet F, Serraf A, et al: Surgical management of neonatal coarctation. *J Thorac Cardiovasc Surg* 109:663-675, 1995.

35. Webber SA, LeBlanc JG, Keeton BR, et al: Pulmonary artery banding is not contraindicated in double inlet left ventricle with transposition and aortic arch obstruction. *Eur J Cardiothorac Surg* 9:515S-520S, 1995.

36. Jensen RA, Williams RG, Laks H, et al: Usefulness of banding of the pulmonary trunk with single ventricle physiology at risk for subaortic obstruction. *Am J Cardiol* 77:1089-1093, 1996.

37. Odim J, Yun J, George B, et al: Staged surgical approach to neonates with aortic obstruction and single ventricle physiology. Presented at the 35th Annual Meeting of the Society of Thoracic Surgeons, San Antonio, Texas, 1999, p 138.

38. Tchervenkov CI, Beland MJ, Latter DA, et al: Norwood operation for univentricular heart with subaortic stenosis in the neonate. *Ann Thorac Surg* 50:822-825, 1990.

39. Rychik J, Murdison KA, Chin AJ, et al: Surgical management of severe aortic outflow obstruction in lesions other than the hypoplastic left heart syndrome: Use of a pulmonary artery to aorta anastomosis. *J Am Coll Cardiol* 18:809S-816S, 1991.

40. Jacobs ML, Rychik J, Murphy JD, et al: Results of Norwood's operation for lesions other than hypoplastic left heart syndrome. *J Thorac Cardiovasc Surg* 110:1555-1562, 1995.

41. Kanter KR, Miller BE, Cuadrado AG, et al: Successful application of the Norwood procedure for infants without hypoplastic left heart syndrome. *Ann Thorac Surg* 59:301-304, 1995.

42. Mosca RS, Hennein HA, Kulik TJ, et al: Modified Norwood operation for single left ventricle and ventriculoarterial discordance: An improved surgical technique. *Ann Thorac Surg* 64:1126-1132, 1997.

43. Brawn WJ, Sethia B, Jagtap R, et al: Univentricular heart with systemic outflow obstruction: Palliation by primary Damus procedure. *Ann Thorac Surg* 59:1441S-1447S, 1995.

44. Chin AJ, Barber G, Helton JG, et al: Fate of the pulmonic valve after proximal pulmonary artery-to-ascending aorta anastomosis for aortic outflow obstruction. *Am J Cardiol* 62:435S-438S, 1988.

45. McElhinney DB, Reddy VM, Silverman NH, et al: Modified Damus-Kaye-Stansel procedure for single ventricle, subaortic stenosis, and arch obstruction in neonates and infants: Midterm results and techniques for avoiding circulatory arrest. *J Thorac Cardiovasc Surg* 114:718S-726S, 1997.

46. Laks H, Gates RN, Elami A, et al: Damus-Stansel-Kaye procedure: Technical modifications. *Ann Thorac Surg* 54:169-172, 1992.

47. Freedom RM, Williams WG, Fowler RS, et al: Tricuspid atresia, transposition of the great arteries, and banded pulmonary artery. *J Thorac Cardiovasc Surg* 80:621-628, 1980.

48. Karl TR, Watterson KG, Sano S, et al: Operations for subaortic stenosis in univentricular hearts [see comments]. *Ann Thorac Surg* 52:420S-428S, 1991.

49. Lacour-Gayet F, Serraf A, Fermont L, et al: Early palliation of univentricular hearts with subaortic stenosis and ventriculoarterial discordance: The arterial switch option. *J Thorac Cardiovasc Surg* 104:1238S-1245S, 1992.

50. Serraf A, Conte S, Lacour-Gayet F, et al: Systemic obstruction in univentricular hearts: Surgical options for neonates. *Ann Thorac Surg* 60:970S-977S, 1995.

51. Frommelt PC, Rocchini AP, Bove EL: Natural history of apical left ventricular to aortic conduits in pediatric patients. *Circulation* 84:213S-218S, 1991.

52. Rothman A, Lang P, Lock JE, et al: Surgical management of subaortic obstruction in single left ventricle and tricuspid atresia. *J Am Coll Cardiol* 10:421S-426S, 1987.

53. Razzouk AJ, Chinnock RE, Gundry SR, et al: Transplantation as a primary treatment for hypoplastic left heart syndrome: Intermediate-term results. *Ann Thorac Surg* 62:1S-7S, 1996.

54. Caspi J, Coles JG, Rabinovich M, et al: Morphological findings contributing to a failed Fontan procedure. Twelve-year experience. *Circulation* 82:177S-182S, 1990.
55. Malcic I, Sauer U, Stern H, et al: The influence of pulmonary artery banding on outcome after the Fontan operation. *J Thorac Cardiovasc Surg* 104:743S-777S, 1992.
56. Seliem M, Muster AJ, Paul MH, et al: Relation between pre-operative left ventricular mass and outcome of the Fontan procedure in patients with tricuspid atresia. *J Am Coll Cardiol* 14:750-755, 1989.
57. Jacobs ML, Rychik J, Rome JJ, et al: Early reduction of the volume work of the single ventricle: The Hemi-Fontan operation. *Ann Thorac Surg* 62:456S-462S, 1996.
58. Douglas WI, Mosca RS, Goldberg CS, et al: The Hemi-Fontan procedure for hypoplastic left heart syndrome. Presented at the 35th Annual Meeting of the Society of Thoracic Surgeons, San Antonio, Texas, 1999, pp 58-59.
59. Lamberti JJ, Spicer RL, Waldman JD, et al: The bidirectional cavopulmonary shunt. *J Thorac Cardiovasc Surg* 100:22S-30S, 1990.
60. McElhinney DB, Marianeschi SM, Reddy VM: Additional pulmonary blood flow with the bidirectional Glenn anastomosis: Does it make a difference? *Ann Thorac Surg* 66:668S-672S, 1998.
61. Freedom RM: The dinosaur and banding of the main pulmonary trunk in the heart with functionally one ventricle and transposition of the great arteries: A saga of evolution and caution. *J Am Coll Cardiol* 10:421-426, 1987.
62. Huddleston CB, Canter CE, Spray TL: Damus-Kaye-Stansel with cavopulmonary connection for single ventricle and subaortic obstruction. *Ann Thorac Surg* 55:339S-346S, 1993.

CHAPTER 10

Early and Medium-term Outcomes After the Fenestrated Fontan Operation

Nancy D. Bridges, M.D.
Associate Professor of Pediatrics, University of Pennsylvania School of
Medicine; Medical Director, Thoracic Organ Transplant and Pulmonary
Hypertension Programs, Children's Hospital of Philadelphia,
Philadelphia, Pennsylvania

In the late 1980s, two groups at opposite ends of the country introduced a new modification to the Fontan operation, to allow a right-to-left shunt at the atrial level. Between 1987 and 1990, Laks et al.[1] operated on 36 patients in whom an "adjustable atrial septal defect" was created at the time of the Fontan operation. Between 1989 and 1990, Castaneda et al.[2] operated on 20 patients in whom a punched "fenestration" was created in the baffle of a lateral tunnel-type Fontan operation. Though the techniques differed, the goals were the same: to avoid the devastating low-output state that was the primary cause of death or takedown after this form of single-ventricle palliation. The specific proposed benefits of these modifications were that cardiac output would be increased, at the expense of oxygenation, with an overall increase in systemic oxygen transport; that pressure in the systemic venous atrium pressure would be reduced; and that these hemodynamic benefits might be associated with improved survival and reduced morbidity. In this review, the extent to which these benefits have been demonstrated in the perioperative period and at follow-up of 2 years or more will be addressed.

There has not been (and likely never will be) a randomized comparison of outcomes after Fontan operation, with and without an atrial-level shunt. The data presented in this review therefore derive from three types of clinical studies. In the first type, comparison is made with contemporary or historical "controls" (i.e., patients undergoing a nonfenestrated Fontan operation). The second type of study referred to is a retrospective series review, with multivariable analysis performed to assess the impact of an intentional right-to-left shunt. Such series must account for improvements in outcome that are independent of the shunt—for example, the impact of a specific surgical technique or of modified ultrafiltration. Finally, data are presented from studies in which the results of acute, transient obstruction of the atrial-level shunt were observed in the cardiac catheterization laboratory.

In examining the impact of baffle fenestration on operative outcomes one must recognize that, as with most surgical interventions for congenital heart disease, outcomes have improved with increased experience. All the reasons for the improved outcomes cannot be identified with certainty, but clearly this improvement has occurred for patients undergoing nonfenestrated Fontan operations as well as those having a baffle fenestration.[3] Furthermore, patients undergoing Fontan operations are heterogeneous with regard to a large number of characteristics that might have an effect on outcome (e.g., cardiac anatomy, age, prior operations), and this limits the validity of comparisons between series from different institutions. Nevertheless, in the most current series, the lowest reported mortality (1 of 55 patients), duration of effusions (none), and mean hospital stay after the Fontan operation (8 days) are in those who have had an intentionally created right-to-left shunt.[4]

EARLY OUTCOMES

The impact of a right-to-left atrial shunt on operative survival, duration of pleural effusions, length of hospital stay, and postoperative hemodynamics has been described. One approach to assessing the impact of baffle fenestration on outcome has been to retrospectively assess risk factors and outcomes in two contemporary groups of patients having operations that were identical except for the presence (n = 91) or absence (n = 56) of a baffle fenestration (Fig 1).[5] The two groups were compared with respect to several preoperative risk factors including pulmonary artery pressure, pulmonary vascular resistance, pulmonary artery distortion, total number of risk factors, and evaluation using a previously developed "risk score."[3] In all respects, patients having an operation with a baffle fenestration were at higher risk based on preoperative characteristics than were those undergoing a nonfenestrated Fontan operation (Fig 2). Nevertheless, survival was virtually identical in the two groups, suggesting that baffle fenestration nul-

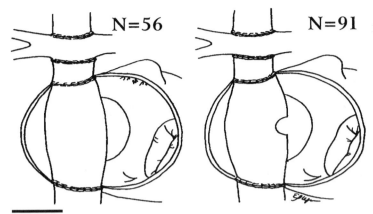

FIGURE 1.
Diagrammatic representation of the type of operations performed in the referenced study (see text). All patients had a lateral tunnel-type of Fontan operation. In 56 patients, the baffle was intact; in 91 patients, a 4-mm hole was punched in the baffle. (Courtesy of Bridges ND, Mayer JE, Lock JE, et al: Effect of baffle fenestration on outcome of the modified Fontan operation. *Circulation* 86:1762-1769, 1992. Used by permission.)

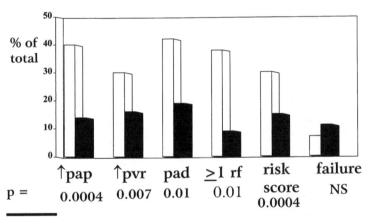

FIGURE 2.
Percent of patients having specific preoperative risk factors. Patients who went on to have an operation with a baffle fenestration are indicated by the *light-colored bars*; patients who went on to have an operation without a fenestrated baffle are indicated by the *dark-colored bars. Abbreviations: pap,* pulmonary artery pressure; *pvr,* pulmonary vascular resistance; *pad,* pulmonary artery distortion; *rf,* risk factor; *NS,* not significant.

lified the impact of those risk factors. In a later review of 500 patients undergoing the Fontan operation, Gentles et al.[6] demonstrated that absence of a baffle fenestration was a very significant ($P = 0.002$) predictor of failure (death or takedown) after a modified Fontan operation. The association between presence of a baf-

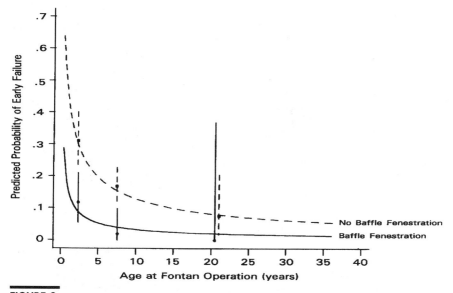

FIGURE 3.
Predicted probability of early failure (death or takedown) after a Fontan operation. Patients without a baffle fenestration have a higher risk of failure; this effect is most important in patients younger than 5 years. (Courtesy of Gentles TL, Mayer JE, Gavreau K, et al: Fontan operation in five hundred consecutive patients: Factors influencing early and late outcome. *J Thorac Cardiovasc Surg* 114:376-391, 1997. Used by permission.)

fle fenestration and improved survival was most marked in the youngest patients (Fig 3).

The same retrospective group comparison cited above also found that the duration of effusions (10.7 days vs. 23.8 days, $P = 0.009$) and the length of hospital stay (13.3 days vs. 21.4 days, $P = 0.005$) were significantly shorter in those having a fenestrated Fontan operation than in those having a nonfenestrated Fontan operation. More recent reports indicate that, with increasing experience, duration of effusions and length of stay have decreased in patients with[4] and without[7] baffle fenestration; however, in contemporary series, patients with a baffle fenestration appear to have a lower risk of pleural effusions and shorter postoperative hospitalizations (Fig 4).

Several authors have examined the impact of acute, transient obstruction of the baffle fenestration or adjustable atrial septal defect on cardiac index and systemic oxygen transport (Table 1).[2,8-11] In all of these series, an open atrial communication resulted in significantly higher cardiac index and systemic oxygen transport. This effect derives at least in part from an increase in preload and ejection fraction, as demonstrated by Kuhn et al.[12]

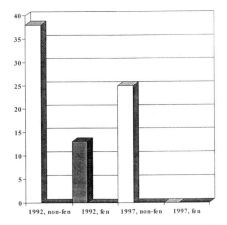

Percent of patients with effusions

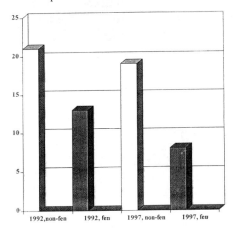

Length of hospital stay

FIGURE 4.
Percent of patients with prolonged pleural effusions and duration of postoperative hospital stay after the Fontan operation. Three series of patients are shown: one from Children's Hospital, Boston (*"1992, fen and non-fen"*); one from Children's Hospital of Philadelphia (*"1997, fen"*), and one from Babies Hospital, New York (*"1997, non-fen"*). The proportion of patients having effusions and the duration of hospitalization have decreased over time, with and without baffle fenestration; however, in each surgical era, those with baffle fenestration are less likely to have effusions and have shorter hospitalizations. *Abbreviations: fen, fenestration; non-fen, nonfenestration.*

Another demonstrated benefit of an atrial communication in the early postoperative period is that of decreased systemic venous pressure. Elevated systemic venous pressure has been identified as a predictor of operative survival after Fontan operation.[6,13,14] The

TABLE 1.

Effect of Baffle Fenestration on Cardiac Index *(CI)* and Systemic Oxygen Transport *(SOT)**

Bridges et al.[2] 1990	n = 17	CI ↑ 36%
Hijazi et al.[8] 1992	n = 14	CI ↑ 23% and SOT ↑ 14%
Mavroudis et al.[9] 1992	n = 13	CI ↑ 12%
Harake et al.[10] 1994	n = 11	CI ↑ 26% and SOT ↑ 9%
Bridges et al.[11] 1995	n = 60	CI ↑ 30% and SOT ↑ 15%

*Results of five studies in which the effect of acute obstruction of the baffle fenestration was observed in the cardiac catheterization laboratory. The Table indicates the increase in CI and SOT that was present with the fenestration open.

postoperative systemic venous pressure was lower among patients having a fenestrated Fontan operation than in those without a fenestration (*P* = 0.004). In addition, the preoperative to postoperative increase in systemic venous pressure was less (5.4 mm Hg vs. 9.3 mm Hg, *P* = 0.0001) among those with a fenestration.[5]

MEDIUM-TERM OUTCOMES

At 2- and 5-year follow-up after a fenestrated Fontan operation, the survival curves remain flat at about 90% (Fig 5).[5,6] Among 60 patients with a fenestrated Fontan operation followed up for an average of 2 years, 83% were in New York Heart Association (NYHA) Class I, with the remainder in Class II.[11] Gentles et al.[6] assessed functional status at a median of 5 years of follow-up among 363 patients who had undergone the Fontan operation, 125 with fenestration; 91% were in NYHA Class I. Baffle fenestration per se was not demonstrated to be associated with improved functional status in that group. However, it has been demonstrated that transient occlusion of the fenestration performed 6 months or more after operation continues to result in a significant increase in systemic venous pressure; and that, regardless of fenestration status, a systemic venous pressure in excess of 16 mm Hg is associated with poor functional status (NYHA Class II or less) at follow-up (*P* = 0.01).[11] Because it is routine to leave the fenestration open if test occlusion results in increased systemic pressure, it seems reasonable to conclude that the fenestration may well be contributing to improved functional status in many of these patients.

Another possible benefit of lower systemic venous pressure is improved cognitive status at follow-up. Wernovsky et al.[15] evaluated the cognitive status of 131 children who had undergone the Fontan operation, using a composite achievement score (CAS). As

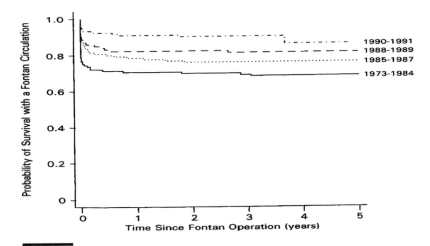

FIGURE 5.
Actuarial survival after the Fontan operation, by surgical era. Survival, especially early survival, has improved with increased experience. The *survival curves* are relatively flat out to 5 years. (Courtesy of Gentles TL, Mayer JE, Gavreau K, et al: Fontan operation in five hundred consecutive patients: Factors influencing early and late outcome. *J Thorac Cardiovasc Surg* 114:376-391, 1997. Used by permission.)

with NYHA Class, fenestration per se did not correlate with a higher composite achievement score, but lower postoperative systemic venous pressure (less than 14 mm Hg) was a predictor of higher scores ($P = 0.02$) in univariate analysis. However, in a multivariate analysis that included characteristics such as prior circulatory arrest and socioeconomic status, elevated right atrial pressure did not retain predictive significance.

The relationship between protein-losing enteropathy and baffle fenestration has been the subject of several reports. In 1994, Mertens et al.[16] described a 29-year-old patient with well-documented protein-losing enteropathy of 3 years' duration, unresponsive to medical therapy. Transcatheter creation of an atrial-level shunt resulted in a decrease in arterial oxygen saturation to 85%, and immediate and sustained resolution of protein-losing enteropathy. Other authors have reported similar experiences.[17,18] It appears that transient improvement can be achieved in virtually all patients in this way, if an adequate communication is created (i.e., one that results in an arterial oxygen saturation in the mid-80s); however, recurrence of symptoms occurs in some. In those with recurrence of protein loss and severe symptoms, heart transplantation has been an effective therapy.

The relationship between baffle fenestration and embolic stroke remains controversial. Embolic stroke is a well-known complication of the nonfenestrated Fontan operation.[19-21] Clearly, in the absence of a right-to-left shunt, the source of embolism must lie on the pulmonary venous side of the Fontan pathway (e.g., a ligated stump of main pulmonary artery), whereas in the presence of a right-to-left shunt, the embolic source may be on either side of the atrial baffle.[22-24] Characteristics that contribute to the increased risk of thromboembolism after Fontan operation probably include increased venous stasis[25] and a hypercoagulable state, which may be related to liver dysfunction (secondary to high systemic venous pressure) or loss of clotting factors resulting from protein-losing enteropathy or chronic pleural effusions.[26] Baffle fenestration decreases the prevalence and severity of some of these characteristics but also provides a pathway for paradoxical embolism. Thus, one might speculate that baffle fenestration would increase, decrease, or have no impact on the incidence of thromboembolic events after the Fontan operation. The largest review of embolic stroke after Fontan operation was that of du Plessis et al.,[27] in which 645 patients undergoing Fontan operations between 1978 and 1993 were reviewed for evidence of embolic stroke. The incidence of embolic stroke in this group was 2.6%, with strokes occurring at an interval of 1 day to 32 months after the operation. No association between baffle fenestration and stroke was demonstrable in this group of patients.

CONCLUSIONS

Incorporation of an atrial-level right-to-left shunt into the Fontan operation is associated with increased cardiac index, increased systemic oxygen transport, increased preload to the systemic ventricle with an associated increase in ejection fraction, and decreased systemic venous pressure. The decrease in systemic venous pressure has been demonstrated both in the immediate postoperative period and at intermediate follow-up, and is almost certainly an important contributor to improved operative survival and medium-term functional status. That baffle fenestration is associated with improved survival can be demonstrated in large series of patients, and this improvement is most evident in those undergoing Fontan operations before the age of 5 years. Baffle fenestration is just one of many modifications of technique introduced since the late 1980s (including the lateral-tunnel approach and the use of modified ultrafiltration) that, along with increased experience and understanding of the patient population, has resulted in almost complete disappearance of operative mortality and morbidity at the time of a Fontan operation.

Many questions remain. The impact of routing of the systemic venous return through an external conduit, and the role of fenestration in this setting remain to be determined. The optimal age at which to perform a Fontan operation remains an open question. The observation that morbidity and mortality are higher in the youngest patients has been made repeatedly in those undergoing a Fontan operation without a fenestration. Use of a fenestration seems to minimize or even eliminate young age as a risk factor in the short-term, but long-term outcomes are only just emerging. Mahle et al.[28] demonstrated that early volume unloading (via a bidirectional cavopulmonary anastomosis or a Fontan operation) is associated with improved exercise capacity at follow-up. This might be seen as an argument to proceed with this type of surgery as early as possible. On the other hand, early imposition of high systemic venous pressure may have a negative effect on cognitive development, and the long-term effect of nonpulsatile, low-pressure, low-volume flow on the pulmonary vascular bed is unknown. Thus, balancing cardiac benefit against the effects on the rest of the child's organ systems will be the key to determining the optimal age for this surgery. Other important questions remain unanswered. Which (if any) fenestrations should be closed—or, if spontaneously closed, should be reopened? Does the relationship between the degree of cyanosis and the increase in cardiac index—and thus, ultimately, the systemic oxygen transport—change over time in a given patient? Do the risks of cyanosis increase with age?

The optimal palliation of the patient with one functional ventricle remains a work in progress. The diversity of opinion with regard to achieving the optimal palliation testifies to the imperfection of our current state of knowledge. At present, the weight of the evidence is in favor of the benefits of an atrial-level shunt in the Fontan operation with regard to minimizing operative mortality and morbidity and improving functional status at medium-term follow-up. The impact of this modification on long-term survival and function remains to be seen.

REFERENCES

1. Laks H, Pearl JM, Haas GS, et al: Partial Fontan: Advantages of an adjustable interatrial communication. *Ann Thorac Surg* 52:1084-1095, 1991.
2. Bridges ND, Lock JE, Castaneda AR: Baffle fenestration with subsequent transcatheter closure: Modification of the Fontan operation for patients at increased risk. *Circulation* 82:1681-1689, 1990.
3. Mayer JE, Bridges ND, Lock JE, et al: Factors associated with marked reduction in mortality for Fontan operations in patients with single ventricle. *J Thorac Cardiovasc Surg* 103:444-452, 1992.
4. Koutlas TC, Gaynor JW, Nicolson SC, et al: Modified ultrafiltration reduces postoperative morbidity after cavopulmonary connection. *Ann Thorac Surg* 64:37-42, 1997.

5. Bridges ND, Mayer JE, Lock JE, et al: Effect of baffle fenestration on outcome of the modified Fontan operation. *Circulation* 86:1762-1769, 1992.

6. Gentles TL, Mayer JE, Gavreau K, et al: Fontan operation in five hundred consecutive patients: Factors influencing early and late outcome. *J Thorac Cardiovasc Surg* 114:376-391, 1997.

7. Hsu DT, Quaegebeur JM, Ing FF, et al: Outcome after single-stage, nonfenestrated Fontan procedure. *Circulation* 969:335S-340S, 1997.

8. Hijazi ZM, Fahey JT, Kleinman CS, et al: Hemodynamic evaluation before and after closure of fenestrated Fontan: An acute study of changes in oxygen delivery. *Circulation* 86:196-202, 1992.

9. Mavroudis C, Zales VR, Backer CL, et al: Fenestrated Fontan with delayed catheter closure: Effects of volume loading and baffle fenestration on cardiac index and oxygen delivery. *Circulation* 86:85S-92S, 1992.

10. Harake B, Kuhn MA, Jarmakani JM, et al: Acute hemodynamic effects of adjustable atrial septal defect closure in the lateral tunnel Fontan procedue. *J Am Coll Cardiol* 23:1671-1676, 1994.

11. Bridges ND, Lock JE, Mayer JE, et al: Cardiac catheterization and test occlusion of the interatrial communication after the fenestrated Fontan operation. *J Am Coll Cardiol* 25:1712-1717, 1995.

12. Kuhn MA, Jarmakani JM, Laks H, et al: Effect of late postoperative atrial septal defect closure on hemodynamic function in patients with a lateral tunnel Fontan procedure. *J Am Coll Cardiol* 26:259-265, 1995.

13. Kirklin JK, Blackstone EH, Kirklin JW, et al: The Fontan operation: Ventricular hypertrophy, age, and date of operation as risk factors. *J Thorac Cardiovasc Surg* 92:1049-1064, 1986.

14. Sanders S, Wright G, Keane J, et al: Clinical and hemodynamic results of the Fontan operation for tricuspid atresia. *Am J Cardiol* 49:1733-1740, 1982.

15. Wernovsky G, Stiles KM, Gauvreau K, et al: Cognitive development following the Fontan operation. *Circulation*, in press.

16. Mertens L, Dumoulin M, Gewilling M: Effect of percutaneous fenestration of the atrial septum on protein-losing enteropathy after the Fontan operation. *Br Heart J* 72:591-592, 1994.

17. Warnes CA, Feldt RH, Hagler DJ: Protein-losing enteropathy after the Fontan operation: Successful treatment by percutaneous fenestration of the atrial septum. *Mayo Clin Proc* 71:378-379, 1996.

18. Rychik J, Rome JJ, Jacobs ML: Late surgical fenestraion for complications after the Fontan procedure. *Circulation* 96:33-36, 1997.

19. Mathews K, Bale J, Clark E, et al: Cerebral infarction complicating Fontan surgery for cyanotic congenital heart disease. *Pediatr Cardiol* 7:161-166, 1986.

20. Driscoll DJ, Offord KP, Feldt RH, et al: Five- to fifteen-year follow-up after Fontan operation. *Circulation* 85:469-496, 1992.

21. Hutto R, Williams J, Maertens P, et al: Cerebellar infarct: Late complication of the Fontan procedure. *Pediatr Neurol* 7:293-295, 1991.

22. Jahangiri M, Ross DB, Redington AN, et al: Thromboembolism after

the Fontan procedure and its modifications. *Ann Thorac Surg* 58:1409-1414, 1994.

23. Rosenthal DN, Friedman AH, Kleinman CS, et al: Thromboembolic complications after Fontan operations. *Circulation* 92:287S-293S, 1995.

24. Wilson DG, Wisheart JD, Stuart AG: Systemic thromboembolism leading to myocardial infarction and stroke after fenestrated total cavopulmonary connection. *Br Heart J* 73:483-485, 1995.

25. Nakazawa M, Nakanishi T, Okuda H, et al: Dynamics of right heart flow in patients after Fontan procedure. *Circulation* 69:306-312, 1984.

26. Cromme-Dijkuis A, Henkens C, Bijlveld C, et al: Coagulation factor abnormalities as possible thrombotic risk factors after Fontan operations. *Lancet* 336:1087-1090, 1990.

27. Du Plessis AJ, Chang AC, Wessel DL, et al: Cerebrovascular accidents following the Fontan operation. *Pediatr Neurol* 12:230-236, 1995.

28. Mahle W, Wernovsky G, Bridges ND, et al: Very early unloading results in improved exercise performance in preadolescents with single ventricle Fontan physiology. *J Am Coll Cardiol*, in press.

CHAPTER 11

The Alternate Recipient List for Heart Transplantation: A Model for Expansion of the Donor Pool

Hillel Laks, M.D.
Professor and Chief, Division of Cardiothoracic Surgery; Director, Heart and Heart-Lung Transplant Program, UCLA Medical Center, Los Angeles, California

Daniel Marelli, M.D.
Assistant Clinical Professor, Division of Cardiothoracic Surgery, UCLA School of Medicine, Los Angeles, California

Every stage of human life except the last is marked by certain defined limits. Old age alone has no precise boundary.

Cicero

Recent trends in United Network for Organ Sharing (UNOS) data show that the number of patients waiting for a heart transplant is increasing consistently, while both the number of transplants and the number of deaths while waiting for a transplant are leveling off.[1] This indicates that the gap between available donors and recipients is widening. Until an alternative to transplantation becomes available, strategies must be developed to expand the donor pool.

The concept of a dual listing system to expand the existing donor pool stems from the hypothesis that certain recipients have specific needs and risk factors that can be used to match them with donor organs that have similar risk factors.[2-4] The aim of the second "alternate" list is to match recipients whose long-term (greater than 5 years) survival is limited with donor organs that have unknown long-term outcome. Such patients have usually been excluded from the option of transplantation because not enough donor organs are available to supply the existing "regular" waiting list. The concept of placing such potential recipients on a second waiting list evolved as a result of some donor hearts being refused because of uncertain long-term outcome despite anticipated excellent immediate posttransplant function.[5]

Intuitively, when a 20-year-old potential recipient is placed on the waiting list for a heart transplant, the expectation is for an organ that can potentially last more than 30 years. In contrast, when a 70-year-old individual is placed on a waiting list, the expectation is for an organ that can potentially last 10 years, because long-term survival of such patients is limited by a process other than graft survival. Thus, the alternate recipient list may offer better survival than does current medical treatment for end-stage congestive heart failure in patients who are, in many instances, turned down for transplantation because of long-term risk.[6]

PATIENTS

Since 1992, 83 patients have been placed on the alternate recipient list. As of 1998, the age criterion for entry was raised from 65 to 70 years of age. All patients are screened for vascular disease and colon cancer in addition to usual guidelines. Reasons for alternate classification are listed in Table 1; age accounted for alternate listing in the largest proportion of the patients.

Sixty-six percent of patients had ischemic cardiomyopathy, 17% had dilated cardiomyopathy, 9% had transplant coronary disease, and 8% had various other cardiomyopathies. Ten patients died while waiting, and 1 patient was removed because of the occurrence of a cancer. As of December 1998, 51 patients have undergone transplantation and 11 patients are currently waiting

---

TABLE 1.

Reasons for Patients to Be Shifted From
the Regular to the Alternate Recipient List

Age (65-74 yr)	87%
Transplant coronary disease + age	12%
Peripheral arterial disease	1%

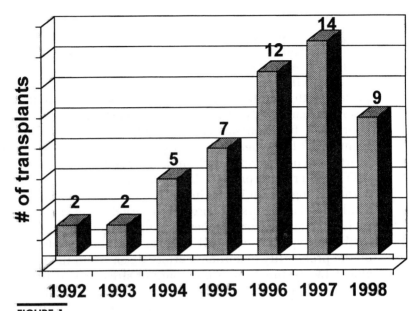

FIGURE 1.
Alternate recipient transplants by year.

(Fig 1). During the same period, 479 standard regularly listed recipients also underwent orthotopic heart transplantation.

RECIPIENT SELECTION

Once accepted for alternate listing, all recipients are informed of the donor-recipient matching process as it will occur and consent is obtained. Alternate recipients are then placed on the UNOS regional waiting list as per national guidelines. Part of the consent process is that they agree to not be upgraded to status I (in hospital, waiting). When a donor heart is considered by a procurement agency, it is offered to regularly listed recipients in the usual order. If it is turned down by our program as well as other programs for regularly listed patients, the donor heart is then reconsidered for the alternate list as a last resort rather than remaining unused. Within our program, the alternate list is kept separate from the regular list. The donor heart is then considered by both the treating surgeon and cardiologist, as well as the patient who, as part of the informed consent, retains the right of refusal, depending on the donor risk factors.

DONOR SELECTION

Donor hearts are routinely assessed with baseline measurements of central venous pressure (CVP) and inotropic support. High inotrope requirement is defined as more than 14 µg/kg/min of dopamine, and high CVP is considered greater than 10 cm H_2O. This information is complemented by echocardiography, which is used to assess left ventricular (LV) contraction and wall thickness, as well as valve function. In general, if LV dysfunction is present, a thyroid hormone infusion is started.[7] More than mild atrioventricular valve dysfunction is considered a reflection of poor heart function unless a correctable anatomical defect is identified.[8] LV hypertrophy is regarded with caution and such hearts are considered only from large-sized donors, particularly if ECG criteria are present. If donors are older than 40 years, a coronary angiogram is obtained.[9] If a coronary angiogram is not available, risk factors for coronary artery disease are considered, including male gender, obesity, hyperlipidemia and diabetes mellitus, hypertension, and tobacco and cocaine abuse. Based on the probability of coronary artery disease and the presence of global LV dysfunction, a dobutamine stress echocardiogram is obtained. If a decision is made to use such a heart, then a coronary artery angiogram is obtained after implant within 14 days. Our own previous results have shown that occurrences of transplant coronary artery disease are not related to preexisting coronary artery disease in older donors.[10]

Donor hearts were selected with the purpose of minimizing organ wastage while ensuring successful outcome as outlined by UNOS. The minimum donor-to-recipient height and weight ratios used were 0.8. Causes of brain death for the donors presented in this series are shown in Figure 2. The most common

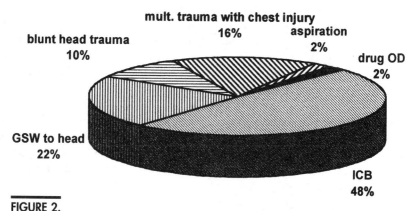

FIGURE 2.
Causes of brain death in donors selected for alternate recipients. *Abbreviations: GSW,* gunshot wound; *ICB,* intracranial bleeding; *OD,* overdose.

TABLE 2.
Isolated Alternate Donor Risk Factors

Reused donor heart	2
Chest trauma/suspected myocardial contusion	4
Extensive substance abuse	3
Small donor, no other matches	3
Hepatitis B	1
Decreased LV function on echocardiogram	1

Abbreviation: LV, left ventricular.

cause was intracranial bleeding. Our donor selection process has been evolving since 1992 as a result of experience and reported results from other groups. Donors were considered alternate because of the presence of one or a combination of several risk factors. Our policy is to consider every available heart for every patient and to weigh donor risk factors against recipient risk factors following the strategy outlined by Young et al.[2] Thus, a donor heart with suspected myocardial contusion and no echocardiogram available may be considered for a small recipient without pulmonary hypertension after sending our retrieval team to visually inspect the heart and measure intracardiac pressures. Such a scenario is ideal in the case of a local donor.

Another consideration was a history of donor substance abuse. This occurred in five instances, three of which were isolated. In the other two, one donor heart had associated dysfunction reflected by high inotrope requirement. The other heart came from an older donor (older than 55 years).

Isolated risk factors were present in 14 donors (Table 2), whereas overlapping multiple risk factors were present in 37 donors (Figs 3 and 4). Older donors were not necessarily considered alternate unless there were associated risk factors. In the case of hepatitis B, surface antibody–positive/antigen-negative donors were considered if core IgM antibody was negative.[11,12] Hepatitis C–positive donor organs were considered after informed consent with the understanding that the estimated risk of seroconversion is 50%, and that the overall risk of chronic liver pathology at 10 years' follow-up is estimated to be about 30% to 40%.[13,14] Ten donor hearts had coronary artery disease without specific segmental wall dysfunction that could be bypassed on the back table using conduits from the recipient. One donor heart required coronary artery angioplasty before retrieval.

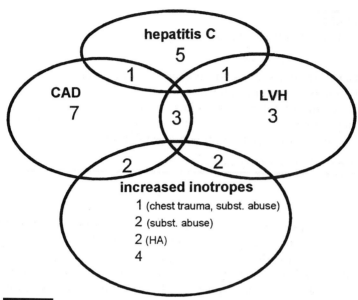

FIGURE 3.
Donor risk factors for alternate recipients. *Abbreviations: CAD*, coronary
artery disease; *LVH*, left ventricular hypertrophy; *HA*, history of cardiac
arrest.

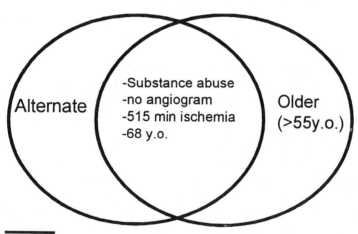

FIGURE 4.
Older donor risk factors.

SURGICAL TECHNIQUE

Donor hearts were preserved using a cold infusion of University of
Wisconsin solution.[15] Infusion pressure is measured after the
ascending aorta is clamped and is limited to 60 mm Hg.[16] Our pro-
tocol emphasizes total infusion time first and volume second.

Thus, donor hearts receive an infusion of 5 to 7 minutes approximating 8 to 10 cc/kg.

During implantation, the recipient's left atrial cuff is vented to remove venous return from the bronchial circulation. On completion of the left atrial anastomosis, a second catheter is advanced into the LV apex so that a cold plasmalyte solution can be infused. This adds to topical cooling of the donor heart and improves de-airing. Similarly, an infusion is also used for the donor right ventricle during completion of the pulmonary and aortic anastomoses.

Reperfusion of the donor heart is started while the inferior vena cava anastomosis is constructed. This consists of leukocyte-depleted warm, aspartate-glutamate enriched blood cardioplegia (Buckberg solution).[17] This is maintained for 3 to 4 minutes after which warm leukocyte-depleted blood is infused for 4 to 5 minutes. Reperfusion aortic root pressure is limited to 50 mm Hg targeting a flow of about 2 to 3 mL/kg/min. The superior vena cava anastomosis is constructed during this time.

Weaning from cardiopulmonary bypass is carried out with dopamine and dobutamine as the first line of inotropic support. This is complemented by nitric oxide inhalation if right ventricular dysfunction or pulmonary hypertension is present. Left atrial pressure is routinely measured in addition to monitoring with a pulmonary artery catheter.

RESULTS

Figure 5 shows the actual number of patients on the alternate list for each year since 1992. As described above, this number decreased in 1998 because of a change in the age limit of our regular list from 65 to 70 years of age. The median waiting time for the 51 patients transplanted to date was 95 days (range, 3-488 days). The median donor age was 46 years (18-68 years). Identical gender match occurred in 75% of cases, and identical ABO match was achieved in 91% of recipients. Average donor-to-recipient height and weight ratios were 1.00 and 1.05, respectively. Donors came from outside our local retrieval area (more than 60 minutes travel time) in 41% of instances. The median postoperative hospital stay was 10 days.

Median follow-up is currently 23 months. Actuarial 4-year survival is 78%, and freedom from transplant coronary disease is 70% (Fig 6). Table 3 lists causes of death as well as recipient and donor risk factors for 10 in-hospital nonsurvivors. One late death occurred at 58 months' follow-up secondary to graft coronary artery disease. Of 11 patients who received hearts that were revascularized, 8 are long-term survivors and graft patency among them is 65%. The longest follow-up in this subgroup is 6 years.

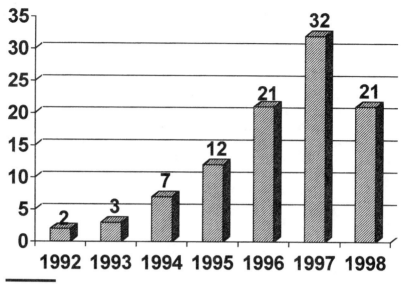

FIGURE 5.
Number of patients listed as alternates. Age level was raised from 65 to 70 years of age between 1997 and 1998.

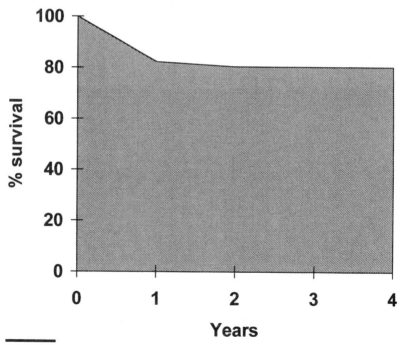

FIGURE 6.
Actuarial survival of alternate recipients 1992-1998.

DISCUSSION

The current gap between donor heart supply and demand is increasing. This, however, does not reflect regional differences in donor availability and practice patterns. This implies that it is conceivable that some donor hearts are not used in one part of the country despite a need in another part of the country. The UNOS system addresses this issue specifically. The alternate recipient list further expands on this concept. As the number of patients waiting for donor hearts increases, and the number of transplants plateaus, it is imperative that every heart available be used. This need will be amplified as the population ages and both donors and recipients get older. The majority of heart transplant recipients are between 18 and 64 years of age. The new UNOS guidelines have already initiated a dual list concept by prioritizing pediatric donors to pediatric recipients. Ultimately, the alternate list will therefore be an adjustable third list that allows for yet another degree of precision in matching donors and recipients.

The mean donor age has been increasing steadily for the last 10 years and is now 30 years.[18] The median donor age in this series was 46 years. This was balanced out by a relatively high donor-to-recipient weight ratio which reflects a selection bias that allowed for use of marginal hearts. More specifically, in many instances hearts were marginal if they had high inotrope requirement or unknown long-term outcome. The former is caused in part by the process of brain death and is potentially reversible. It represents a threat to the immediate postoperative survival. It was therefore mitigated by minimizing other risk factors according to the model of Young et al.,[2] as well as by using improved preservation methods. The latter being irreversible, as in the example of a hepatitis C–positive donor, can be mitigated by matching the organ to recipients with similarly unknown long-term outcome. In this instance, there is no threat to early postoperative function.

The survival rate achieved in the current follow-up is comparable to our regularly listed recipients. One can imagine that this will not be sustained after 7 or 8 years. It is important to note that in all the instances of early graft failure (Table 3), the donor risk factors included age greater than 45 years, coronary artery disease, LV hypertrophy, and long distance. This has caused us to review our experience with LV hypertrophy and to be more conservative with this risk factor.[19] The other seven early deaths were recipient related.

One unexpected observation in the data presented is that the number of alternate heart transplants performed decreased in the last year by 30% (5 transplants). Parallel to this, the total number of heart transplants performed by our program decreased by 5% (5). This is in contradistinction to our track record in the last 3

TABLE 3.
Causes of Early Mortality

Patient	Year	Survival (days)	Cause of Death	Recipient Risks	Donor Risks
OG	1994	40	Lung infection	67 y/o, hx of coccidioidomycosis	57 y/o, CAD
RK	1994	11	Graft failure	66 y/o	55 y/o, CAD LVH, distant
IS	1994	2	Hyperacute rejection	68 y/o, high PRAs	LV dysfunction, hx of arrest, female > male
GG	1995	149	MSOF, sepsis	62 y/o, retransplant, renal insufficiency	Donor/recipient: Wt = 0.75, Ht = 0.96
CO	1996	6	Graft failure	67 y/o DM, previous CABG	CAD, LVH, distant
BS	1997	60	MSOF, sepsis	38 y/o, obesity, retransplant, renal insufficiency, Hep C, DM	LVH, Hep C
WP	1997	174	MSOF, sepsis, sig-moid volvulus	66 y/o DM	Substance abuse, hx arrest
RM	1998	34	MSOF, pneumonia	68 y/o, previous CABG	58 y/o, substance abuse
JB	1998	4	Arrhythmia	69 y/o	49 y/o, CAD, LVH, distant, substance abuse
OS	1998	51	MSOF	51 y/o, retransplant ¥ 2	Hep C

Abbreviations: y/o, years old; *hx,* history; *CAD,* coronary artery disease; *LVH,* left ventricular hypertrophy; *PRAs,* panel reactive antibodies; *MSOF,* multisystem organ failure; *DM,* diabetes mellitus; *CABG,* coronary artery bypass grafting; *Hep,* hepatitis.

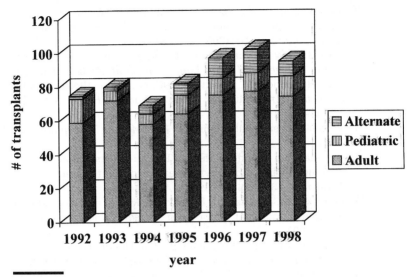

FIGURE 7.
Heart transplants performed at UCLA.

years that shows an increase in number of transplants (alternate and regular) despite a decreasing trend in registry data (Fig 7).[18] One possible explanation for the decrease in the number of transplants is the change in our alternate list criteria that raised the age bar from 65 to 70 years. This had the effect of reducing the number of patients on the alternate list, resulting in fewer available patients to match to an available alternate donor. Such hearts, therefore, may have been unused.

The alternate list was initiated to give certain patients the opportunity to receive a heart transplant that they otherwise would not have. The model that was created is, to our knowledge, the first formal attempt to match donor risk to recipient risk. It also appears to demonstrate that using two adult recipient lists based on patient needs and donor risks may actually increase the total number of transplants performed. It is possible that in the future, as the need for donors increases, the alternate list age bar will be decreased as long-term results of this model become available. This strategy will then be complemented by other options such as destination therapy with mechanical support.

REFERENCES

1. United Network for Organ Sharing Web site. Available at: http://www.unos.org. Accessed February 1, 1999.
2. Young J, Naftel D, Bourge R, et al: Matching the heart donor and heart transplant recipient. *J Heart Lung Transplant* 13:353-365, 1994.

3. Jeevanandam V, Furukawa S, Prendergast TW, et al: Standard criteria for an acceptable donor heart are restricting heart transplantation. *Ann Thorac Surg* 62:1268-1275, 1996.
4. Laks H: Only optimal donors should be accepted for heart transplantation: Antagonist. *J Heart Lung Transplant* 14:1043-1046, 1995.
5. Laks H, School FG, Drinkwater DC, et al: The alternate recipient list for heart transplantation: Does it work? *J Heart Lung Transplant* 16:735-742, 1997
6. Kesten S: Is survival important? *J Heart Lung Transplant* 17:651-653, 1998.
7. Jeevanandam V, Todd B, Regillo T, et al: Reversal of donor myocardial dysfunction by triiodothyronine replacement therapy. *J Heart Lung Transplant* 13:681-687, 1994.
8. Boucek MM, Mathis CM, Kanakriyeh MS, et al: Donor shortage: Use of the dysfunctional donor heart. *J Heart Lung Transplant* 12:186S-190S, 1993.
9. Livi U, Bortolotti U, Lucianai GB, et al: Donor shortage in heart transplantation. *J Thorac Cardiovasc Surg* 107:1346-1355, 1994.
10. Drinkwater DC, Laks H, Blitz A, et al: Outcomes of patients undergoing transplantation with older donor hearts. *J Heart Lung Transplant* 15:684-691, 1996.
11. Wachs ME, Amend WJ, Ascher NL, et al: The risk of transmission of hepatitis B from HbsAg(-), HbcAb(+), HBIgM(-) organ donors. *Transplantation* 59:230-234, 1995.
12. Uemoto S, Sugiyama K, Marusawa H, et al: Transmission of hepatitis B virus from hepatitis B core antibody-positive donors in living related liver transplants. *Transplantation* 65:494-499, 1998.
13. Ali MK, Light JA, Barhyte DY, et al: Donor hepatitis C virus does not adversely affect short-term outcomes in HCV+ recipients in renal transplantation. *Transplantation* 66:1694-1697, 1998.
14. Lake KD, Smith CI, LaForest SK, et al: Outcomes of hepatitis C positive (HCV+) heart transplant recipients. *Transplant Proc* 29:581-582, 1997.
15. Stein DG, Drinkwater DC, Laks H, et al: Cardiac preservation in patients undergoing transplantation. *J Thorac Cardiovasc Surg* 102:657-665, 1991.
16. Ihnken K, Morita K, Buckberg GD: New approaches to blood cardioplegic delivery to reduce hemodilution and cardioplegic overdose. *J Card Surg* 9:26-36, 1994.
17. Pearl JM, Drinkwater DC, Laks H, et al: Leukocyte-depleted reperfusion of transplanted human hearts: A randomized, double-blind clinical trial. *J Heart Lung Transplant* 11:1082-1092, 1992.
18. Hosenpud JD, Bennett LE, Keck BM, et al: The registry of the International Society for Heart and Lung Transplantation: Fifteenth official report—1998. *J Heart Lung Transplant* 17:656-668, 1998.
19. Marelli D, Laks H, Moriguchi J, et al: Is the use of donor hearts with left ventricular hypertrophy acceptable? *J Heart Lung Transplant* 18:87, 1999.

Index

A

B

M